Improving America's Diet and Health

From Recommendations to Action

A report of the Committee on
Dietary Guidelines Implementation

Food and Nutrition Board
Institute of Medicine

Paul R. Thomas, *Editor*

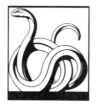

NATIONAL ACADEMY PRESS
Washington, D.C. 1991

NATIONAL ACADEMY PRESS • 2101 Constitution Avenue, N.W. • Washington, D.C. 20418

NOTICE: The project that is the subject of this report was approved by the Governing Board of the National Research Council, whose members are drawn from the councils of the National Academy of Sciences, the National Academy of Engineering, and the Institute of Medicine. The members of the committee responsible for the report were chosen for their special competencies and with regard for appropriate balance. This report has been reviewed by a group other than the authors according to procedures approved by a Report Review Committee consisting of members of the National Academy of Sciences, the National Academy of Engineering, and the Institute of Medicine.

The Institute of Medicine was established in 1970 by the National Academy of Sciences to enlist distinguished members of the appropriate professions in the examination of policy matters pertaining to the health of the public. In this, the Institute acts under both the Academy's 1863 congressional charter responsibility to be an adviser to the federal government and its own initiative in identifying issues of medical care, research, and education. Dr. Samuel O. Thier is president of the Institute of Medicine.

This study was supported by the Henry J. Kaiser Family Foundation through Grant No. 87-4338 and by the National Cancer Institute, National Institutes of Health, U.S. Department of Health and Human Services, through Contract No. N01-CN-85072.

Library of Congress Cataloging-in-Publication Data

Institute of Medicine (U.S.). Committee on Dietary Guidelines Implementation.
     Improving America's diet and health: from recommendations to action /
a report of the Committee on Dietary Guidelines Implementation, Food and
Nutrition Board, Institute of Medicine; Paul R. Thomas, editor.
          p. cm.
     Includes bibliographical references.
     Includes index.
     ISBN 0-309-04139-2
     1. Diet—Standards—United States. 2. Nutrition policy—United States.
     3. Health. I. Title.
     [DNLM: 1. Diet. 2. Health. 3. Nutrition. 4. Risk Factors.
          QU 145 I593i]
RA784.I57 1991
363.8'0973—dc20
DNLM/DLC
for Library of Congress
                                                                    91-7471
                                                                       CIP

Printed in the United States of America

The serpent has been a symbol of long life, healing, and knowledge among almost all cultures and religions since the beginning of recorded history. The image adopted as a logotype by the Institute of Medicine is based on a relief carving from ancient Greece, now held by the Staatlichemuseen in Berlin.

COMMITTEE ON DIETARY GUIDELINES IMPLEMENTATION

EDWARD N. BRANDT, JR. (*Chairman*), Health Sciences Center, University of Oklahoma, Oklahoma City, Oklahoma

NORMAN M. KAPLAN (*Vice Chairman*), University of Texas Southwestern Medical Center, Dallas, Texas

STANLEY ARONSON, Brown University, Providence, Rhode Island

LORELEI DiSOGRA, Nutrition and Cancer Prevention Program, California Public Health Foundation, Sacramento, California

JANICE M. DODDS, School of Public Health, University of North Carolina, Chapel Hill, North Carolina

CHARLES DWYER, Graduate School of Education, University of Pennsylvania, Philadelphia, Pennsylvania

JOHANNA T. DWYER, Frances Stern Nutrition Center, New England Medical Center Hospital, Boston, Massachusetts

JOHN W. FARQUHAR, Center for Research in Disease Prevention, Stanford University School of Medicine, Palo Alto, California

JOAN D. GUSSOW, Department of Nutrition Education, Teachers College, Columbia University, New York, New York

D. MARK HEGSTED, New England Regional Primate Center, Harvard Medical School, Southborough, Massachusetts

H. O. KUNKEL, College of Agriculture and Life Sciences, Texas A&M University, College Station, Texas

LESTER LAVE, Graduate School of Industrial Administration, Carnegie-Mellon University, Pittsburgh, Pennsylvania

BERNARD J. LISKA, Department of Food Science, Purdue University, West Lafayette, Indiana

BEATRICE MARKS, Ketchum Public Relations, New York, New York

ODONNA MATHEWS, Giant Food, Inc., Landover, Maryland

RICHARD E. PETTY, Department of Psychology, Ohio State University, Columbus, Ohio

BONITA WYSE, College of Family Life, Utah State University, Logan, Utah

Committee on Diet and Health Liaison Members

HENRY BLACKBURN, School of Public Health, University of Minnesota, Minneapolis, Minnesota

DONALD B. McCORMICK, Department of Biochemistry, Emory University School of Medicine, Atlanta, Georgia

ANTHONY B. MILLER, Department of Preventive Medicine & Biostatistics, University of Toronto, Toronto, Ontario, Canada

Staff

PAUL R. THOMAS, *Project Director* (from January 1990; formerly Program Officer)
LENORA MORAGNE, *Project Director* (to December 1989)
FRANCES M. PETER, *Editor* (to August 1990)
MARIAN M. F. MILLSTONE, *Research Assistant* (to July 1990)
GERALDINE KENNEDO, *Senior Secretary* (from April 1990)
MARION RAMSEY ROBERTS, *Senior Secretary* (from January to December 1989)

FOOD AND NUTRITION BOARD

Staff

CATHERINE E. WOTEKI, *Director* (from April 1990)

ALVIN G. LAZEN, *Interim Director* (from September 1989 to April 1990)

SUSHMA PALMER, *Director* (to August 1989; consultant to committee from September 1989 to February 1990)

FRANCES M. PETER, *Deputy Director* (to August 1990)

SHIRLEY ASH, *Financial Specialist*

UTE S. HAYMAN, *Administrative Assistant*

Preface

In late 1987, the Henry J. Kaiser Family Foundation and the National Cancer Institute commissioned the National Academy of Sciences to develop a comprehensive plan to implement the scientific consensus that has emerged on dietary guidelines as a means to improve the health of Americans and to assess the possible consequences of implementing the plan. A committee was formed in the Institute of Medicine's Food and Nutrition Board (FNB) to accomplish the project's two major goals:

• propose detailed strategies and options for the implementation of dietary guidelines by government agencies at all levels; by professionals in the nutrition, medical, and allied health fields; by educational institutions and those who provide nutrition information to the public; and by certain segments of the private sector, including institutions concerned with mass feeding; and

• to the extent possible, examine the potential benefits and costs of implementing dietary guidelines.

This report is closely related to an earlier report of the FNB entitled *Diet and Health: Implications for Reducing Chronic Disease Risk* (NRC, 1989). That report provided a comprehensive review of the relationships of dietary patterns and nutrient intake to the risk of diet-related chronic diseases that affect Americans; it included nine recommendations for maintaining health. In the present report, the Committee on Dietary Guidelines Implementation proposes a series of strategies and actions to put those recommendations into action.

However, the strategies and actions are sufficiently general to be applied as well to several sets of dietary recommendations developed during the 1980s.

The intended audience for this report is the many people who share some responsibility for implementing dietary recommendations in the United States. Examples of implementors include public- and private-sector policymakers, supermarket managers, restaurant owners, food writers, the entire nutrition community, and deans of schools of higher education.

FORMATION OF COMMITTEE AND COMMITTEE PROCEDURES

The 17-member interdisciplinary Committee on Dietary Guidelines Implementation was appointed in early 1988. In addition, there were three liaison members from the Committee on Diet and Health and from the FNB. Collectively, the membership provided expertise in nutrition science and education, dietetics, epidemiology, preventive medicine, public health, public policy, food production, food retailing, food marketing, food safety, community nutrition intervention strategies, social and behavioral psychology, public relations, medicine, medical science administration, and cost-benefit analysis. In preparing this report, the committee drew on its own considerable resources as well as the diverse experiences of agencies, organizations, consultants, and other experts working to improve eating habits in the United States.

The committee met 10 times during the course of the study. Early in its work, it obtained and reviewed many materials, including descriptions of efforts to promote more healthful eating patterns and influence consumer behavior. In addition, a public meeting was convened in July 1988 as a forum for representatives of the food industry, professional societies, voluntary organizations, advocacy groups, and interested consumers. The committee also held several workshops to obtain more detailed information from individuals whose experiences in implementing guidelines on diet and health were believed to be particularly important.

Four task forces composed of committee members were established to develop implementation strategies and actions for specific broad sectors of society: (1) the public sector (legislative and executive branches of governments); (2) the private sector (areas as diverse as segments of the food industry to the work site); (3) health-care professionals (including nutritionists, physicians, and nurses, both as practitioners and as members of associations); and (4) public education (defined broadly to include the many settings in which learning occurs). In developing recommendations for consideration by the full committee, each task force studied what had been done and what was currently being undertaken to implement dietary recommendations in these sectors. Important incentives, constraints, and barriers to implementation for these societal sectors were also identified.

As a result of information-gathering efforts and activities within the task forces, the committee was able to define its approach to the task, to learn what has and has not worked in changing dietary habits, and to identify gaps in the knowledge base. The committee then developed strategies and actions for implementation by specific sectors of society as well as three broad strategies for implementation based largely on the commonalities identified among the four sectors. In response to the second part of its charge, the committee attempted to make some assessments of the costs and benefits to the United States of implementing the committee's recommendations; it was unsuccessful in these efforts because of the paucity of data. Although different parts of this report were drafted by different groups, it represents the consensus of the entire committee rather than the views of individual members or task forces. As is to be expected in any committee endeavor, not every member may agree with every specific point. However, all members agree that the statements represent the consensus view.

This report contains nine chapters. Chapter 1 provides a summary of the entire report and the committee's principal strategies for implementing dietary recommendations. The product of the deliberations of the task forces and a presentation of background and assessments of critical elements of the study appear in Chapters 2 through 8. In Chapter 9, the committee identifies the research needed to develop more successful implementation initiatives.

SCOPE AND LIMITATIONS OF REPORT

In a public policy report such as this, it is important to make clear its scope and limitations. This report does not provide a blueprint for carrying out a coordinated, national effort to improve dietary patterns in the United States. Our charge was simply too broad (one sympathetic, anonymous reviewer described it as "Herculean" in scope), our size too small, and our time too short to develop very specific recommendations for the behavior of large, diverse, and complex societal sectors. In addition, it was difficult to reach agreement among all participants on basic elements of a national nutrition policy and how its activities should be coordinated and prioritized. In retrospect, the extreme difficulty of our task should not have been surprising. Our committee simply reflected the larger society in holding many different views about what should be done to improve dietary patterns in this country and how it should be done. Because the biomedical and social science literature provide few data on which to base specific recommendations, opinion and professional judgment prevail, inevitably producing conflict.

Our recommendations are therefore general by design and default. To the extent that they call for changing existing programs and practices, implementation will be uncomfortable or difficult, will take considerable time, and in many cases will require new and redirected financial resources. For example, our recommendations for mass media campaigns to enhance public awareness of dietary recommendations and for the expansion of nutrition education at all levels may seem impractical at a time of high budget deficits when funding for such initiatives will be difficult to obtain. We have tried to make our recommendations practical and attainable with an eye toward the realities of the contemporary political, economic, and social environments, but our primary consideration in selecting them was that they are likely, in our judgment, to improve American diets.

Each recommendation of this committee has implications which, depending on one's perspective, can be perceived as desirable or undesirable. For example, our recommendation that guidelines be developed for book publishers to enable them to provide consistent and authoritative information on dietary recommendations might be applauded by some and interpreted by others as a recommendation for a censorship board. This disagreement illustrates the fact that our political and social leanings and biases affect how we view recommendations to encourage or push us to behave in certain ways. Recommendations which may be considered by some to be protective or in the interests of public health may be seen by others as paternalistic, intrusive, and a violation of rights or infringing on civil liberties, freedom of choice, and free enterprise. We believe that our recommendations are detailed enough to provide adequate direction for implementing dietary recommendations, yet general enough so as to encourage public debate in deciding how to carry them out.

Rather than laying out a very specific plan for implementation, this report provides reasonably detailed recommendations that in the committee's judgment should be the basis of efforts to improve the diet and health of Americans. Many recommendations have specified or obvious outcomes so that progress in achieving them can be measured. The best index indicating that the committee's recommendations have been reached will be evidence from surveys (e.g., the Nationwide Food Consumption Survey and the National Health and Nutrition Examination Survey) of populationwide dietary changes to meet dietary recommendations.

A public policy report in which recommendations are made less on the basis of experimental data and more on considered professional judgment will receive extensive review and criticism. This we welcome. Having largely met the challenge of achieving scientific consensus on the composition and components of healthy diets, it is now time to face the even greater challenge of encouraging and enabling people to eat better. To the extent that this report leads to greater efforts to face and meet that challenge through discussion, debate, new initiatives, and extensions of important initiatives already in progress, the committee considers its efforts a success.

ACKNOWLEDGMENTS

The committee thanks the many individuals and organizations who contributed to this report by providing important information and by serving as consultants, advisers, informal reviewers, and presenters at workshops. They include Emerita N. Alcantara, National Dairy Council; American Dietetic Association; American Health Foundation; American Heart Association; American Society for Clinical Nutrition; Elaine Bratic Arkin, Health Communication; Ronald Baker, C & B Feedyards; Stephen Balsam, Food and Nutrition Service (FNS), U.S. Department of Agriculture (USDA); Amy Barr, *McCall's* magazine; Clement Bezold, Institute for Alternative Futures; Susan T. Borra, Food Marketing Institute (FMI); Marilyn Burkart, National League for Nursing; Marion Burros, *New York Times*; C. Wayne Callaway, George Washington University; Charles J. Carey, National Food Processors Association; Carol Carlson, ARA Services; Linda Cleveland, Human Nutrition Information Service (HNIS), USDA; Victor Cohn, *The Washington Post*; Gerald F. Combs, Agricultural Research Service, USDA; Frances Cronin, HNIS, USDA; Callie Crossley, ABC News; Patricia Daniels, FNS, USDA; Eileen DeLeeuw, Utah State University; Arnold E. Denton, Campbell Soup Company; Robert Dorfman, Emeritus Professor of Economics, Harvard University; Adam Drewnowski, University of Michigan; Mary Egan, Egg Nutrition Center; Chet England, Burger King Corporation; Carol Fletcher, Grocery Manufacturers of America, Inc.; Florida Department of Health and Rehabilitative Services; Allan L. Forbes, Food and Drug Administration (FDA), U.S. Department of Health and Human Services (DHHS); John Francis, National Live Stock and Meat Board; Ardyth H. Gillespie, Cornell University; Mary T. Goodwin, Montgomery County (Maryland) Department of Health; Dottie Griffith, *Dallas Morning News*; Joan Guberman, American College Health Association; Timothy M. Hammonds, FMI; James T. Heimbach, HNIS, USDA; Elisabet Helsing, World Health Organization; Thomas A. Hodgson, National Center for Health Statistics, DHHS; Hilarie Hoting, American Meat Institute; Michael Jacobson, Center for Science in the Public Interest; Marsha D. Kelly, National Council of State Boards of Nursing, Inc.; Chor-San Khoo, Campbell Soup Company; John LaRosa, George Washington University; Bryan R. Luce, Battelle Human Affairs Research Centers; Barbara Luke, Board on Agriculture, National Research Council; J. Michael McGinnis, Office of Disease Prevention and Health Promotion (ODPHP), DHHS; Elaine McLaughlin, United Fresh Fruit and Vegetable Association; Linda D. Meyers, ODPHP, DHHS; Nancy Milio, University of North Carolina at Chapel Hill; Kathryn Montgomery, University of California at Los Angeles; Marion Nestle, New York University; New York State Department of Corrections; William D. Novelli, Porter/Novelli; Grace L. Ostenso, U.S. House of Representatives, Committee on Science, Space and Technology; Lynn Parker, Food Research and Action Center; Betty B. Peterkin, HNIS, USDA (retired); Donna V. Porter, Congressional Research Service; Claire Regan, National Restaurant Association; James Rotherham, U.S. House of Representatives, Committee on Agriculture; Sarah Setton, The Sugar Association, Inc.; Becky Smith, Association for the Advancement of Health Education; Elwood W. Speckman, National Dairy Council; Marilyn G. Stephenson, FDA, DHHS; Tennessee Child Nutrition Program; George W. Tressel, National Science Foundation; Nancy J. Tucker, Produce Marketing Association, Inc.; U.S. Department of Defense; Michael J. Wargo, U.S. General Accounting Office; Susan Welsh, HNIS, USDA; Michael White, National Heart, Lung, and Blood Institute of the National Institutes of Health; and Donna M. Woolcott, University of Guelph. Our thanks go as well to those anonymous individuals who formally reviewed the penultimate draft of this report and provided extremely helpful comments and suggestions. Of course, the committee assumes full responsibility for the contents of this report and the opinions expressed in it.

Completion of this report would not have been possible without the efforts of the Food and Nutrition Board staff, particularly Paul R. Thomas, as well as Catherine E. Woteki, Sushma Palmer, Frances Peter, and Lenora Moragne; research assistance by Marian M.F. Millstone; administrative assistance from Geraldine Kennedo, Marion Ramsey Roberts, and Dionis Gaines; and copy editing by Michael K. Hayes and Wallace K. Waterfall. The committee also expresses its thanks and appreciation to the members of the FNB who gave their time and expertise to the review of this manuscript. Special recognition and thanks are also due to Sarah Samuels and Alvin Tarlov of the Kaiser

Family Foundation and to Luise Light and Suzanne Haynes of the National Cancer Institute for their encouragement and support.

Finally, the committee would like to thank the staff of the National Academy Press, particularly Sally Stanfield, Richard E. Morris, and Scott F. Lubeck, for their assistance in publishing this report. Special acknowledgment is due to Samuel O. Thier and Enriqueta C. Bond of the Institute of Medicine as well as Alvin G. Lazen and John E. Burris of the Commission on Life Sciences for their expert advice, oversight, and constant encouragement throughout the course of this study.

EDWARD N. BRANDT, JR.
Chairman
Committee on Dietary Guidelines
Implementation

REFERENCE

NRC (National Research Council). 1989. Diet and Health: Implications for Reducing Chronic Disease Risk. Report of the Committee on Diet and Health, Food and Nutrition Board, Commission on Life Sciences. National Academy Press, Washington, D.C. 749 pp.

Contents

9   Directions for Research   210

Appendix A: Dietary Recommendations   215

Appendix B: Summary of Committee's
     Major Recommendations   218

Acronyms   227

Index   229

1

Summary

D IETARY RECOMMENDATIONS for the U.S. population have been promulgated for almost a century. Early dietary guidance was directed mainly at the avoidance of deficiency diseases, with little attention given to reducing the risk of chronic conditions other than obesity. However, there have been substantial advances in the past 25 years in understanding the relation of diet to health. As a result, consensus has developed about the role of diet in the etiology and prevention of chronic diseases. The National Research Council report, *Diet and Health: Implications for Reducing Chronic Disease Risk* (NRC, 1989; hereinafter referred to as the *Diet and Health* report) and *The Surgeon General's Report on Nutrition and Health* (DHHS, 1988) provide authoritative reviews of the evidence relating dietary factors to health and disease and make clear that there is now broad agreement on the overall nature of dietary modifications to reduce the risk of diet-related chronic diseases.

The main challenge no longer is to determine what eating patterns to recommend to the public (although, admittedly, there is more to be learned), but also how to inform and encourage an entire population to eat so as to improve its chance for a healthier life. There has been an increasing recognition that simply issuing and disseminating recommendations is insufficient to produce change in most people's eating behaviors. Many federal and state programs exist to implement the federal government's dietary guidelines. Also, there are persistent efforts by the private sector to produce and publicize food products that help people to meet various recommendations. How-

1

ever, there remains a clear need for comprehensive and coordinated actions to improve America's diet and health.

The Committee on Dietary Guidelines Implementation was convened in 1988 under the auspices of the Food and Nutrition Board (FNB) of the Institute of Medicine to address this widely felt need. In this report, the committee promotes the recommendations of the *Diet and Health* report. These recommendations are well suited for implementation because they are the most comprehensive and authoritative currently available and have been established by an eminent group of biomedical scientists based on a comprehensive evaluation of the scientific evidence linking nutrient intake, food intake, and dietary patterns with risks of developing many chronic degenerative diseases. In addition, the *Diet and Health* recommendations specify quantitative targets (e.g., limit fat intake to 30% or less of calories) and are presented in a priority order that reflects their likely impact on public health; they will be reviewed regularly and revised as needed to incorporate new findings. All of these qualities facilitate their interpretation and translation into specific strategies and actions for implementation.

Nevertheless, the committee's goals, strategies, and actions for implementation are qualitative and apply equally well to the recommendations in the *Diet and Health* report, *The Surgeon General's Report on Nutrition and Health* (DHHS, 1988), and the *Dietary Guidelines for Americans* report of the U.S. Departments of Agriculture and Health and Human Services (USDA/DHHS, 1990) (see Appendix A for all 3 sets of recommendations). The third serves as the basis for nutrition policies of the federal government. The term *dietary recommendations* is used throughout this report to refer as a group to these three documents of dietary guidance. This committee's strategies and actions proposed for implementation also apply to most of the dietary guidelines issued by expert groups that focus on specific diseases (e.g., guidelines issued by the American Heart Association and the National Cancer Institute), because they are similar to those of the FNB, Surgeon General, and USDA/DHHS.

The committee believes that the United States should move toward adopting a single set of dietary recommendations to communicate and promote. One set of recommendations should reduce confusion and provide implementors with a common focus for their activities.

PLACING DIETARY RECOMMENDATIONS IN PERSPECTIVE

Although the focus of this report is on improving dietary patterns, the committee emphasizes that diet is only one important determinant of health and well-being. Various personal behaviors (e.g., refraining from smoking and abuse of drugs, engaging in regular exercise, and taking care to avoid accidents) and other factors (e.g., family history of disease, access to health-care services, and the state of the environment) are also strongly linked to risks of disease and should not be neglected in health promotion programs by an overemphasis on diet. Healthful dietary behaviors and other ways of life will improve the health of many people but will not guarantee good health or long life for any person.

The committee hopes that implementation initiatives undertaken in response to the recommendations in this report will be linked with other health-promoting practices whenever possible. A long-term commitment to implementation by promoting incremental changes is more likely to be successful than are drastic, one-shot efforts. Because the food system and public responses to new dietary patterns change slowly, a realistic time frame for implementation will be measured in years rather than months.

ISSUES IN IMPLEMENTING DIETARY RECOMMENDATIONS

The primary issue facing the committee was to determine how the U.S. population could be mobilized to improve its eating patterns to reduce the prevalence of diet-related chronic diseases. This goal will be met in the following ways:

• enhancing awareness, understanding, and acceptance of dietary recommendations;
• creating legislative, regulatory, commercial, and educational environments supportive of the recommendations; and
• improving the availability of foods and meals that facilitate implementation of the recommendations.

The general tactics for increasing the prevalence of healthful eating patterns can be divided into three classes:

• *Altering the food supply*—by *subtraction* (e.g., reducing the fat in meat and cheese), *addition* (e.g., appropriate fortification of foods with nutrients), and *substitution* (e.g., replacing some of the fat in margarine with water).
• *Altering the food acquisition environment*—by providing *more food choices* that help consumers meet dietary recommendations, *better information* (e.g., more complete and interpretable product labeling), *advice at points of purchase* (e.g., tags indicating a good nutrition buy in supermarkets or cafeterias), and *more options* for selecting health-

ful diets (e.g, better food choices in vending machines and restaurants).

- *Altering nutrition education*—by *changing the message mix* (e.g., presenting consistent messages in education programs, advertisements for products, and public service announcements) and by *broadening exposure to formal and nonformal nutrition education* (e.g., mandating education on dietary recommendations from kindergarten through grade 12, in health-care facilities, and in medical schools).

Although common sense suggests that desirable dietary changes will most likely occur when all these components are made to be mutually reinforcing, there is insufficient research on their individual effectiveness or how they can best be assembled into a package.

As related in Chapter 3, there is evidence that some people have already adopted eating patterns that are consistent with dietary recommendations. Throughout the United States, for example, per-capita consumption of fresh fruits and vegetables, breakfast cereals, and other grains has increased, and consumption of whole milk is declining while that of low-fat milk is increasing. Many consumers report that they use less salt and fat in food preparation. But other changes in consumption patterns, such as increasing intake of high-fat cheeses and frozen desserts, fats and oils, snack foods, candy, and some alcoholic beverages, do not appear to be consistent with good nutrition principles.

As is the case with changing dietary patterns, recent changes in consumer attitudes and beliefs about food and nutrition provide cause for both optimism and concern. Overall, there is a general trend toward recognition of the important role that diet plays in disease prevention, but surveys indicate that many people lack both the detailed knowledge and the skills needed to act effectively on this information. Consumers often seem unable to translate the recommendations into food choices or to assess the suitability and composition of their own diets in comparison with the recommendations.

This country's increasing attention to promoting healthy eating patterns and providing advice on how to achieve dietary change can be credited to many developments. These include the preparation of dietary recommendations by experts and the efforts of the private sector to reduce the fat and sodium content of many traditional food products and to provide voluntary nutrition information programs. In addition, the media, recognizing that nutrition sells, have been instrumental in calling the public's attention to dietary recommendations. These efforts, although commendable, have been fragmented, not necessarily consistent, and thus far insufficient to promote large-scale dietary modification. Most people in the United States do not choose diets that conform to dietary recommendations, and current efforts to communicate these recommendations seem to benefit primarily those who are educated and of higher socioeconomic status.

How can the barriers to dietary change be overcome and the public become motivated to adopt healthier diets? Promoters of dietary change need to acknowledge that eating is often social and fun. The committee does not wish to have people focus on health alone in deciding what to eat but, rather, to encourage them to modify their eating behaviors in ways that are both healthful and pleasurable. Promotion of dietary change among currently healthy people may be especially challenging, because the immediate physical and psychological benefits may not be apparent and the appeal is most commonly made on the grounds of potential future well-being.

Although the committee recognizes the difficulty of modifying eating behavior, its extensive review of current theory and practice in Chapter 3 suggests that it is possible to modify food preferences and eating patterns in this country. Some of the factors affecting food choices are difficult to modify (e.g., inherent taste preferences and household income), but other factors such as cultural and social norms (which largely determine what, when, where, how much, and how quickly food is to be eaten), knowledge of and beliefs about food, skills at food selection and preparation, and availability of health-promoting foods are more subject to modification. Initiatives to promote dietary change tend to be most effective when they identify means to help people (1) make the information personally relevant, (2) integrate the information into existing belief structures, (3) acquire new skills and self-perceptions, and (4) select situations that will help them translate newly acquired attitudes into behaviors that become habitual. Research in schools, at work sites, and in communities indicates that certain theory-based intervention programs can produce significant reductions in risk factors for diet-related diseases. It seems reasonable to infer that new national programs to promote the adoption of dietary recommendations by individuals, together with policies that increase the availability of health-promoting foods, will lead to improved dietary patterns.

THE TASKS AND THE PARTICIPANTS IN IMPLEMENTATION

Implementation begins with the conveyance of dietary recommendations to the U.S. population in a language and format that is relevant and comprehensible to the majority of people of all backgrounds, cultures, languages, and interests. The information provided must identify the components of a healthful diet. Proper interpretation of dietary recommendations is essential if implementors—including food planners, cooks, educators, policymakers, curriculum designers, the private sector, and health-care professionals, as well as individuals— are to use them consistently and successfully in a wide variety of contexts. Chapter 4 interprets the nine dietary recommendations of the *Diet and Health* report and provides general guidance for their use in selecting and preparing foods and constructing healthful diets. The guidance is also relevant to the implementation of most recent sets of dietary guidelines.

Both individual and societal actions are needed to encourage and enable Americans to alter their food consumption practices in more healthful directions. Individuals have the responsibility to seek out and use information to improve their eating habits. Sectors of society—including governments, the private sector, health-care professionals, and educators—have responsibilities to facilitate the adoption of better diets by increasing the availability and accessibility of health-promoting foods and using their considerable resources to make such foods easily identifiable (e.g., improved nutrition labeling and nutrition education), economical, and appealing. Society also has an obligation to ensure that food choices over which individual consumers rarely have control (e.g., meals served in institutional cafeterias, on airplanes, or at various social events) are, whenever possible, sufficiently varied so that those who wish to eat in accordance with the principles of dietary recommendations are able to do so.

The committee began its work by imagining a wide range of strategies for modifying eating behavior. To the extent possible, each of these was examined in terms of such criteria as history of effectiveness, affordability, political feasibility, public acceptability, and legal and ethical considerations. Together, these criteria served as the basis for selecting intervention strategies and actions that in the committee's judgment are likely to be successful. The committee concluded that its recommended strategies and actions could not be put in any order of importance or priority because they are diverse in scope, each requiring different levels of resources and participation from various societal sectors, and they all are important and should be carried out simultaneously.

Much of the committee's work was done by four task forces, each focusing on specific societal sectors: public, private, health-care professions, and public education. These groupings were an effective mechanism for identifying the main interventions that have been attempted and for recommending those that might be undertaken. The recommendations of these task forces clearly overlap; they are presented in Chapters 5 through 8 and summarized below.

Public Sector

This sector includes governments at all levels—the executive, legislative, and judicial branches at the federal, state, and local levels. Governments promote implementation of dietary recommendations through direct efforts of legislation and rule-making; provision of information and education; awarding of research and demonstration grants; intramural research, education, and extension programs; food assistance and farm programs; their own vast meal service functions; and in acting as role models by providing examples of implementation in government facilities, by government officials, and at government-funded events. The public sector can also encourage this effort indirectly by setting an agenda for the implementation of various strategies, opening communication with the private sector and voluntary organizations, and coordinating implementation efforts. The five strategies and associated actions developed for the public sector are described in Chapter 5 and summarized below.

1. Improve coordination of federal efforts to implement dietary recommendations. Although the federal government has done much to encourage Americans to eat well, there is no governmentwide nutrition policy that provides a coherent blueprint for fostering healthful dietary patterns. The committee recommends that the executive branch establish a comprehensive coordinating mechanism to promote the implementation of dietary recommendations by all government agencies with responsibilities in food and nutrition. The U.S. Congress and state legislative bodies also need to be active in implementation by developing and passing relevant legislation and by overseeing agency activities.

2. Alter federal food assistance, food safety, nutrition, and farm subsidy, tariff, and trade programs (e.g., the Food Stamp Program, School Lunch Program, and Commodity Distribution Program) that directly influence the food consumed by many of the nation's schoolchildren, elderly people, residents on Indian reservations, and most other Americans to encourage the consumption of diets that meet dietary recommendations.

3. Change laws, regulations, and agency practices that have an appreciable but indirect impact on consumer dietary choices or that will make more foods available to support nutritionally desirable diets. Examples include nutrition labeling of foods, food standards of identity, dairy price supports, quality grading of meat, and descriptors for ground beef.

4. Enable government feeding facilities to serve as models to private food services and help people to meet dietary recommendations.

These facilities include U.S. Department of Veterans Affairs hospital cafeterias; U.S. Department of Defense dining halls, hospitals, and clinics; eating facilities in jails; government cafeterias; and establishments where official meal functions are held.

5. Develop a comprehensive research, monitoring, and evaluation plan to achieve a better understanding of the factors that motivate people to modify their eating habits and to monitor the progress toward implementation of dietary recommendations. The National Nutrition Monitoring System will need to be improved, expanded, and provided with adequate resources.

The committee believes that successful implementation of dietary recommendations by the public sector requires adherence to the following principles: (1) provide information and education; (2) ensure freedom of choice by providing adequate choice at reasonable prices whenever possible; (3) foster long-term commitment and incremental approaches to dietary change to minimize disruption of food preferences; (4) facilitate access to health-promoting foods; (5) present healthful eating in a context of total health promotion; (6) involve all who have some stake in planning and implementing actions; (7) ensure that healthful diets are appealing and convenient and entail the fewest disruptions to current food preferences and life-styles; and (8) encourage the incorporation of health-promoting foods in food programs. These principles also served the committee in devising many of its recommendations for other societal sectors.

Private Sector

In this report, the private sector is defined broadly to include producers of several major commodities (fruits and vegetables, grains and legumes, dairy products, meat, poultry, fish and seafood, and eggs); food manufacturers, processors, and retailers; food service establishments (restaurants, fast-service food establishments, and institutional food-service providers); and work sites (cafeterias and vending machines in office buildings and factories). The two strategies and associated actions developed for the private sector are described in Chapter 6 and summarized below.

1. Promote dietary recommendations and motivate consumers to use them in selecting and preparing foods and in developing healthful dietary patterns. This can be done, for example, by using the methods of public relations and advertising and by providing a variety of user-friendly consumer information programs and materials at retail outlets, food-service establishments, and work sites (e.g., infor-

mation on the nutritional value of specific products at points of purchase). The private sector should initiate and participate in collaborative efforts with other societal sectors to develop consumer education and information programs and materials. It should also continue to contribute to efforts to improve the nutrition labeling of food.

2. Increase the availability of a wide variety of appealing foods that help consumers meet dietary recommendations. New food products are being developed—and traditional ones modified, usually by reducing their total fat, saturated fat, sodium, or sugar content or by increasing their fiber content—in response to scientific consensus about diet and health relationships, consumer interest, and the availability of new technologies and ingredients. It is now easier to select health-promoting meals in many food-service establishments. The private sector should also contribute to efforts to revise or develop food quality criteria (such as standards of identity and grading), pricing structures, and food product descriptors to promote the production of more nutritionally desirable food products. In addition, this sector should fund or conduct surveys on consumer attitudes, knowledge, and practices regarding food and nutrition issues to receive more guidance on how to improve their products and campaigns to encourage healthful eating patterns.

Although there are obvious barriers, there are also many incentives for the private sector to assist consumers in implementing dietary recommendations. The hinderances include the costs of new product research, development, and promotion as well as lack of knowledge or practical guidance on how to make changes in the food supply; the latter is partly due to the fact that many companies do not employ registered dietitians or nutritionists and that chefs and food-service personnel often do not have sufficient background or training in nutrition or in recipe or menu modification. Yet many incentives for the private sector exist to help implement dietary recommendations. These include the potential for an enhanced image and increased product sales, and new and repeat business by increasing customer satisfaction and loyalty.

Health-Care Professionals

People are looking more and more to nutritionists, physicians, nurses, health educators, and other health-care professionals to provide clear information on the links between dietary patterns and risks of disease as well as practical guidelines for eating in ways that meet dietary recommendations. In addition, health-care professionals have renewed interest in preventive over reparative practices. This group performs multiple roles in implementing dietary recommendations beyond their roles as educators and advisers. As organizers, they initiate or contribute to community programs to improve nutrition, and as investigators, they gain new knowledge about diet and disease relationships and the factors that govern behavioral change. The three strategies and associated actions developed for health-care professionals are described in Chapter 7 and summarized below.

1. Raise the level of knowledge among all health-care professionals about food, nutrition, and the relationships between diet and health. The committee recommends (1) establishment of an identifiable program within the faculty of every health-care professional school to plan and develop a research and education agenda in human nutrition; (2) establishment of a program within the U.S. Public Health Service to support the training of faculty in nutrition; (3) development of curricular materials emphasizing dietary recommendations; and (4) encouragement of licensing and certification bodies to require a demonstration of knowledge of nutrition for students in health-care professional schools before graduation.

2. Contribute to efforts that will lead to health-promoting dietary changes for health-care professionals, their clients, and the general population. Health-care professionals should integrate nutrition information into their contacts with clients and patients. They and their professional associations should take advantage of opportunities to disseminate sound nutrition advice through the media; provide guidance to regulatory and legislative bodies concerned with the establishment of policies governing the production, harvesting, processing, preservation, distribution, and marketing of food products; and distribute practical information such as menus, recipes, and ideas for health promotion initiatives to private and public providers of meals.

3. Encourage the public and private sectors to intensify research on the relationships between food, nutrition, and health and on the means to use this knowledge to promote the consumption of healthful diets. The results of such research will enable health-care professionals to provide up-to-date nutrition advice and counseling in more effective ways.

Major barriers to the implementation of dietary recommendations by many health-care professionals include inadequate time and compensation to provide the kinds of nutrition guidance that individuals may desire or need, the perception that many people lack interest in eating better and that they do not follow recommended diets, inadequate knowledge and skills needed to teach people how to improve their diets, and inadequate preparation for their new and expanding roles as promoters of good nutrition. Fortunately, programs established by foundations, voluntary organizations, governments, and other groups are attempting to help health-care professionals prepare for their expanded roles.

Education of the Public

The committee divided education of the public into three categories based on the settings in which learning is assumed to occur: *formal* (in schools), *nonformal* (organized teaching and learning events that occur, for example, in hospitals, community centers, and clinics), and *informal* (the almost infinite variety of educational experiences that include preparing dinner, watching product advertising on television, and reading a newspaper article). Educators face difficulties in helping consumers to eat in ways that meet dietary recommendations in an extensive, complicated, and confusing information environment that includes tens of thousands of food products from which to choose. Success is most likely to be achieved if emphasis is placed on the importance of developing healthful dietary patterns rather than teaching consumers about nutrients whose presence in food products can be individually concentrated or diluted in ways to make these products appear more desirable.

The six strategies and associated actions proposed for education of the public are described in Chapter 8 and summarized below.

1. Ensure that consistent educational messages about dietary recommendations reach the public. This can occur if leaders of various national groups concerned with health develop a series of common educational initiatives to implement the recommendations. Materials prepared by these groups should be reviewed prior to publication to ensure consistency and compatibility with dietary recommendations. In addition, broad guidelines should be developed that publishers could use to convey consistent and authoritative information on dietary recommendations. The educational materials from various food industry sources made available to schoolteachers should also be reviewed and evaluated.

2. Incorporate principles, concepts, and skills training that support dietary recommendations in all levels of schooling. For example, a model curriculum for teaching food skills, nutrition, and health from kindergarten through grade 12 should be developed and should include teacher-tested lessons. Institutions of higher learning should offer a nutrition course for interested students. Additional actions to achieve this strategy include (i) mandating the inclusion of a food skills, nutrition, and health course in teacher preparation programs

in each state; (ii) reviving the successful Nutrition Education and Training (NET) Program, administered by the U.S. Department of Agriculture, which linked classroom teaching about nutrition with the lunchroom and trained school food service personnel to prepare meals based on the lessons they had learned; and (iii) offering each student in grades 7 through college a periodic computer analysis of his or her diet and a professional evaluation of how the student's food habits conform to dietary recommendations.

3. Ensure that children in child-care programs receive nutritious meals served in an environment that takes account of the importance of food to children's physical and emotional well-being. An interdisciplinary task force of experts could develop national recommendations for legislation, regulations, and standards, as well as education and training guidelines for professionals and the public to ensure achievement of this recommendation.

4. Enhance consumers' knowledge and skills needed to meet dietary recommendations through appropriate food selection and preparation. This would entail the development of a consumer manual that outlines strategies for influencing local food providers and appropriate others to increase the availability of nutritionally-desirable foods. Also, the preparation of an inexpensive, continually updatable foods data bank would provide consumers, food planners, and others with the nutritional content, composition, and production/processing histories of the products available to them.

5. Establish systems for designing, implementing, and maintaining community-based interventions to improve dietary patterns. Relevant professional organizations should work to engage community leaders in the development of community-based programs that promote dietary recommendations. Schools of higher learning in various regions of the United States should be encouraged to develop programs to educate and update individuals in the skills they need to play key roles in community nutrition education projects.

6. Enlist the media to help decrease consumer confusion and increase the knowledge and skills that will motivate and equip consumers to make health-promoting dietary choices. This can be done in part through social marketing campaigns and by coordinating media activities to promote healthful eating. In addition, committees should be appointed to review whether television food advertising aimed at children should be regulated and to examine the utility of national entertainment television as a community organizing tool that can be used to enhance efforts of local health agencies in encouraging appropriate dietary changes.

PRINCIPAL IMPLEMENTATION STRATEGIES

In addition to developing recommendations for implementation by individual sectors of society, the committee derived three principal strategies to form the basis for furthering the implementation of dietary recommendations across all sectors. In the committee's judgment, these principal implementation strategies collectively offer the best promise of success in bringing about desirable dietary changes on a national level. Although the committee acknowledges that each of them is already being implemented to some extent, it believes that progress can and should be accelerated.

1. *Governments and health-care professionals must become more active as policymakers, role models, and agenda setters in implementing dietary recommendations.* As described above, governments at the federal, state, and local levels have many opportunities to encourage, empower, and enable more people to improve the quality of their diets. The opportunities come largely from their control over the spending of public funds and, at least as important, by their ability to set public policy (e.g., enact legislation and revise laws, standards, regulations, and rules) and to bring public attention and interest to issues they deem important. The federal government, for example, is reviewing or revising its policies on food labeling, standards of identity and grading of food, and distribution of surplus food commodities as a result of knowledge and concerns about diet and health. The committee believes that greater interest and action by governments in promoting healthy life-styles will contribute greatly to improving dietary patterns in the United States—particularly if top government leaders become involved (e.g., the President, Congress, governors, and mayors) and if governments take opportunities to participate in implementation efforts developed by other societal sectors.

Health-care professionals, who are viewed by the public as credible authorities on matters of health and disease, also have many opportunities to encourage and instruct people on how to improve their dietary habits and other health-related behaviors. As described earlier, health-care professionals, working alone and collectively through their societies and associations, should use their knowledge of diet and disease connections and their practical applications to improve their own diets and the diets of their clients. Health-care professionals should also be active in creating or encouraging initiatives to improve dietary patterns in their communities. Finally, they can create opportunities to contribute to local, state, and national policies that regulate access to nutritionally desirable foods and to the establishment of social environments that encourage healthy eating.

2. *Improve the nutrition knowledge of the public and increase the opportunities to practice good nutrition.* If individuals are to be encouraged to take responsibility for adopting and maintaining healthy behaviors, they need information (to identify problem behaviors and how to improve them), motivation (to make the changes), and supportive environments (to maintain the changes).

Because food habits are formed to a great extent during childhood, incorporating the principles of food, nutrition, and health into preschool, elementary school, and secondary school education—and providing children with health-promoting meals in those settings—offer major opportunities to encourage the development of healthful eating patterns. These efforts must begin in preschool and child-care settings, where an increasing number of children are receiving care. In addition, colleges and institutions of higher learning should make available to students a course in nutrition or healthy life-styles. Health-care professionals also need adequate training about the role of diet in disease prevention and treatment and the practical applications of dietary recommendations at their educational institutions and in continuing education programs. Even schools that train chefs and cooks should place emphasis on dietary recommendations and how they can be used to prepare nutritious and health-promoting meals.

Expected improvements in the nutrition labeling of foods provide further justification for comprehensive nutrition education programs. Although updated nutrition labels will supply important information to interested consumers, the information alone is not sufficiently complete for making wise dietary choices and constructing healthful diets. An important component of nutrition education programs will be to help consumers understand the proper uses and inherent limitations of food labels in planning healthful diets.

In addition to formal schooling, there are many other opportunities that can be used to inform consumers on the connections between diet and health and how to develop healthy food habits. Work sites provide unique opportunities for health and nutrition education because the programs are convenient to employees and the availability of social support from coworkers for changes in behavior is often great. Many food retailers and food-service establishments can provide nutrition information and literature to their customers as well as important point-of-purchase information near specific products.

The communications media (e.g., television, radio, and popular magazines) exert powerful influences on people's lives. Organized campaigns to disseminate, explain, and promote dietary recommendations through a variety of media offer great potential for improving eating patterns in the United States. Funds for campaigns will have to come from both the public and private sectors. Such campaigns should be directed to the general public as well as to selected subgroups of the population, including schoolchildren, disadvantaged and minority populations, the media itself, health-care professionals, and opinion leaders (e.g., celebrities and public officials). In designing media campaigns, emphasis should be placed not simply on developing public service messages and documentaries but also on modifying the contents of programs so that both participants and plots support good eating habits. If media campaigns are to be successful, however, they will have to be coordinated with community-based health promotion efforts.

Local communities provide people with education, work, family and social life, and important services, and can therefore be a powerful force that shapes people's life-styles and health behaviors. Therefore, community-based interventions and programs have an enormous potential for improving dietary patterns in the United States. Effective community-based health promotion programs consist of multiple interventions directed at multiple levels (e.g., individuals, small groups, organizations, and entire communities). Interventions include the development of nutrition education programs at such places as work sites, schools, places of worship, and city or county health departments as well as the provision of information on diet and health at these sites and in local supermarkets, restaurants, government offices, offices of health-care professionals, and many other locations. Communities could, for example, establish nutrition and health committees to generate and coordinate local activities. Membership in the committees should be broad and include interested citizens, health-care professionals, government officials, and local businessmen.

3. *Increase the availability of health-promoting food.* The U.S. food supply is both abundant in variety and high in quality. This is particularly evident in supermarkets in most areas, where people who wish to eat according to dietary recommendations can select from a wide variety of high-quality vegetables and fruits; whole-grain breads and cereals; legumes; lean meats, poultry, and fish; low- or nonfat dairy products; and foods low in added salt and sugar. The private sector has been modifying many traditional products to make them more nutritionally desirable as technology permits and as marketing opportunities are identified.

Yet successful implementation of dietary recommendations will require that consumers have greater access to health-promoting foods on those occasions when they are unable or unwilling to prepare it.

The industries and personnel who provide and prepare food in hospitals, at work-site cafeterias, at airlines, and in vending machines should examine their policies and practices to determine how they can conform to the principles of dietary recommendations. The same applies to food services and food programs administered by federal, state, and local governments, including U.S. Department of Veterans Affairs medical centers, General Services Administration cafeterias, and the school lunch and elderly feeding programs. Restaurants, cafeterias, and fast-service food establishments have special responsibilities to promote better eating by providing foods and meals, prepared in attractive and tasty ways, that help people to meet dietary recommendations. Institutional food-service suppliers should reevaluate their inventories so they are able to supply eating establishments with an increased variety of health-promoting foods.

·It may be especially difficult for people in some parts of the country (e.g., very small towns, rural areas, and economically deprived areas of cities) to eat in ways that meet dietary recommendations if they must depend heavily on small nearby supermarkets or grocery stores for their food purchases. These retailers have a special responsibility to stock as great a variety of nutritionally desirable foods as they are able at reasonable prices.

DIRECTIONS FOR RESEARCH

Continued research is essential to establish a better base for designing cost-effective, efficient, and effective implementation strategies and for assessing their costs and benefits. The committee identified six broad areas of research in which more activity is required to achieve these goals. They are described in Chapter 9 and are identified below.

1. Improve methods to characterize what people actually eat, especially over long periods during which dietary patterns change.

2. Increase understanding of the existing and potential determinants of dietary change and how this knowledge can be used to promote more healthful eating behaviors.

3. Continue research to develop new food products and modify both the production and processing of traditional products to help consumers more easily meet dietary recommendations.

4. Review and improve government and private-sector policies that directly and indirectly affect the availability of particular foods and the promotion of healthful dietary patterns.

5. Determine how implementors of dietary recommendations at

all levels (e.g., supermarket managers, physicians, and high school health teachers) can more effectively teach the basis of the recommendations and motivate people to follow them.

6. Investigate the costs and benefits of implementing dietary recommendations as proposed by this committee and by others.

LESSONS LEARNED AND PROCESS FOR FUTURE

A turning point in nutrition history has been reached. Wide-scale consensus now exists on the types of dietary patterns that promote health and reduce the risks of common degenerative diseases, and at the same time there is great public interest in diet, nutrition, and health issues. Many millions of Americans have modified their diets in desirable directions as a result of past and current implementation efforts. Yet considerable challenges lie ahead if the majority of the U.S. population is to eat in ways that conform to dietary recommendations. Achievement of this overall objective will require unprecedented levels of collaboration among the many entities involved in providing nutrition information, education, and food to the public.

It is time to accelerate efforts to improve America's diet and health.

REFERENCES

DHHS (U.S. Department of Health and Human Services). 1988. The Surgeon General's Report on Nutrition and Health. DHHS (PHS) Publ. No. 88-50210. Public Health Service, U.S. Department of Health and Human Services. U.S. Government Printing Office, Washington, D.C. 727 pp.

NRC (National Research Council). 1989. Diet and Health: Implications for Reducing Chronic Disease Risk. Report of the Committee on Diet and Health, Food and Nutrition Board, Commission on Life Sciences. National Academy Press, Washington, D.C. 749 pp.

USDA/DHHS (U.S. Department of Agriculture/U.S. Department of Health and Human Services). 1990. Nutrition and Your Health. Dietary Guidelines for Americans, 3rd ed. Home and Garden Bulletin No. 232. U.S. Department of Agriculture/ U.S. Department of Health and Human Services, Washington, D.C. 28 pp.

2

Introduction

THE CENTRAL CHARGE to the Committee on Dietary Guidelines Implementation of the Food and Nutrition Board (FNB) was to determine how to implement most effectively the consensus that has emerged regarding the dietary advice that will best promote the public's health.

For almost a century, dietary guidelines for the U.S. population have been promulgated by the federal government and other bodies (Haughton et al., 1987; U.S. Congress, Senate, 1909). Because the maintenance of human health requires the ingestion of nutrients found in food, much of the early dietary advice focused on urging people to eat the kinds and amounts of foods needed to avoid nutrient deficiency diseases. Little attention was given to developing dietary guidance intended to reduce the risk of chronic degenerative disease because there was, until recently, little supporting evidence—other than that linking excess energy intake to obesity—to support such guidelines.

Over the past 25 years, however, substantial advances have been made in understanding the relationships among dietary patterns, food and nutrient intakes, and the etiology and pathogenesis of many chronic degenerative diseases. The roles of diet in health promotion and risk reduction and in the prevention and control of specific diet-related diseases have now been characterized. Beginning in the early 1960s, various sets of dietary guidelines intended to help the population reduce its risk of certain chronic degenerative diseases began to be widely disseminated. These are described and compared in the FNB's

18

report, *Diet and Health: Implications for Reducing Chronic Disease Risk* (NRC, 1989c) (hereinafter referred to as the *Diet and Health* report). The federal government in particular has issued several important sets of dietary guidelines since the late 1970s. Congress, the legislative branch of government, held hearings on dietary patterns and health in the late 1960s and early 1970s that led to the promulgation of *Dietary Goals for the United States* (U.S. Congress, Senate, 1977a,b), suggesting an eating pattern very similar to that later recommended in the *Diet and Health* report. The impetus then passed to the executive branch of government. In 1979, for example, the Surgeon General of the United States published *Healthy People: the Surgeon General's Report on Health Promotion and Disease Prevention* (DHEW, 1979), a landmark document wherein the federal government explicitly recognized the importance of nutrition as a major influence on the nation's health. The following year, this recognition was expanded by the inclusion of 17 specific nutrition objectives in the report *Promoting Health/Preventing Disease: Objectives for the Nation* (DHHS, 1980). Interest in nutrition as a major component of disease prevention and health maintenance was further emphasized with the publication in 1980 of *Nutrition and Your Health: Dietary Guidelines for Americans* (USDA/DHHS, 1980)—a joint project of the U.S. Departments of Agriculture (USDA) and Health and Human Services (DHHS) that became the basis for federal nutrition policies.

Until recently, efforts to act on new understandings about diet and health were focused primarily on achieving consensus among scientists on the appropriateness of certain dietary guidelines and on publicizing various, somewhat different sets of guidelines. These efforts culminated in the issuance of *The Surgeon General's Report on Nutrition and Health* in 1988 (DHHS, 1988) and the FNB's *Diet and Health* report in 1989 (NRC, 1989c). Together, these authoritative reviews of the evidence relating dietary factors to health and disease make it clear that there is now wide-scale consensus in the United States—and in the international nutrition community—on the overall nature of the dietary modifications needed to reduce the risk of diet-related chronic diseases. Indeed, there is a striking level of agreement at this time among dietary guidelines in the United States and those in other industrialized countries around the world (NRC, 1989c).

In this report, the committee promotes the recommendations of the *Diet and Health* report because they are well suited for implementation. These comprehensive recommendations will be reviewed regularly and revised as needed to incorporate new findings. In addition, they specify quantitative targets (e.g., limit fat intake to 30% or less of calories) and are presented in a priority order that reflects their likely impact on public health. These qualities facilitate their interpretation and translation into specific strategies and actions for implementation and facilitate evaluations of the success of these initiatives.

This committee believes that dietary guidelines used as the basis for nutrition policy in the United States should be as quantitative as possible. Therefore, the federal government's progress, albeit slow, in quantifying its dietary guidelines is to be applauded. Examples of quantitation include the following:

• The report *Healthy People 2000: National Health Promotion and Disease Prevention Objectives* issued by DHHS (1990) recommends that average total fat intake among people age 2 and older be no more than 30% of calories and that saturated fat intake not exceed 10% of calories. It also advises the daily consumption of five or more servings of vegetables, fruits, and legumes and six or more servings of grain products.

• The population panel of the National Cholesterol Education Program (NCEP, 1990) recommends that "healthy Americans" beginning at age 2 consume less than 10% of total calories from saturated fatty acids, an average of 30% or less of calories from total fat, and less than 300 mg of cholesterol per day.

• The text of the recently issued 3rd edition of the USDA/DHHS booklet, *Nutrition and Your Health: Dietary Guidelines for Americans*, recommends that total fat intake in the diets of adults not exceed 30% of calories and that saturated fat intake be less than 10% of calories (USDA/DHHS, 1990). The report notes that this recommendation does not apply to children below age 2. The report also recommends that adults eat daily at least three servings of vegetables, two servings of fruits, and six servings of grain products, and that pregnant women or women trying to conceive avoid alcoholic beverages.

• The USDA food guide, "A Pattern for Daily Food Choices," suggests 6-11 servings per day of breads, cereals, and other grain products; 2-4 servings of fruits; and 3-5 servings of vegetables (including dry peas and beans) (USDA, 1989).

The committee's strategies and actions for implementation are qualitative and therefore apply equally well to the recommendations in the *Diet and Health* report, *The Surgeon General's Report on Nutrition and Health* (DHHS, 1988), and *Dietary Guidelines for Americans* (USDA/ DHHS, 1990) (see Appendix A for all three sets of recommendations). Thus, the term *dietary recommendations* is used throughout this report to refer as a group to these three sets of guidelines. The committee's recommended implementation strategies and actions also apply to most or all of the disease-specific dietary guidelines issued by expert groups (e.g., by the American Heart Association and the National Cancer Institute), because they are similar to those of the FNB, the Surgeon General, and USDA/DHHS. However, the committee believes that the United States should move toward adopting a single set of dietary recommendations to communicate and promote. One set of recommendations should reduce confusion and provide implementors with a common focus for their activities.

PLACING DIETARY RECOMMENDATIONS IN PERSPECTIVE

Although this report focuses on improving dietary patterns, the committee emphasizes that diet is only one important determinant of health and well-being. Various personal behaviors (e.g., refraining from smoking and abuse of drugs, engaging in regular exercise, and taking care to avoid accidents) and other factors (e.g., family history of disease, access to health-care services, and the state of the environment) are also strongly linked to risks of disease and should not be neglected in health promotion programs by an overemphasis on diet. Healthful dietary patterns and life-styles will improve the health of many people but will not guarantee good health or long life for any person.

The committee hopes that implementation initiatives undertaken in response to the recommendations in this report will be linked with other health-promoting practices whenever possible. A long-term commitment to implementation by promoting incremental changes is more likely to be successful than are drastic, one-shot efforts. Because the food system and public responses to new dietary patterns change slowly, a realistic time frame for implementation will be measured in years rather than months.

FROM GUIDANCE TO IMPLEMENTATION

Consensus on dietary guidance is an important advance; however, guidelines cannot be effective until a coordinated effort is made to teach consumers how to interpret and apply them and to assist people in overcoming the difficulties in trying to change their eating behaviors. But the many questions about what should be done, and by whom, and where the effort should be focused have not yet been addressed systematically. This lack is partly a consequence of a common, though incorrect, assumption that once there is widespread awareness of dietary guidelines, most people will adopt and implement them on their own. In this report, the committee addresses these and other questions and presents the components of a comprehensive plan to implement dietary recommendations. Although most people in the United States do not choose diets that conform to all the dietary recommendations, some people have changed their diets in recent years for what they report to be health reasons (FMI, 1990). The changes in public attitude and food consumption reported in Chapter 3 are often attributed to public awareness of various sets of dietary guidelines, but it is clear this is not the entire explanation.

Although smoking, as an addictive habit, is very different from eating, the long and continuing effort to reduce cigarette smoking may offer some useful analogies to the task of changing eating habits. The antismoking effort has involved alterations in the physical environment (by restricting areas in which smoking can occur); positive examples of nonsmoking by highly visible individuals (e.g., physicians and politicians); promotion of tobacco avoidance in public and private education; and assistance to smokers who want to quit. The public and private sectors have devoted effort and money to the cause. Of equal importance, however, may have been the common purpose shown at most levels of government (with continued tobacco subsidies a notable exception) and the vast effort expended by health-oriented voluntary groups such as the American Cancer Society, the American Heart Association, the American Lung Association, and Action on Smoking and Health. Even greater commitments of money, time, political will, and other resources will likely be needed to improve the nation's eating patterns.

IMPLEMENTATION AND THE POOR

This report is directed to the majority of the U.S. population, which enjoys secure access to food. There is another segment of the population, however, that has tragically little food security and has uncertain or inconsistent access to a wholesome, nutritious food supply. This group includes people who are poor or homeless and people who are disadvantaged and dependent because of disease or other reasons (Mayer, 1990; Stoto et al., 1990). Their diets may not supply adequate calories and may be low in vitamins and minerals but high in total fat, saturated fat, cholesterol, and sodium. Alcohol abuse may also affect some people in this group. The nutritional status of the poor and disadvantaged can be further compounded by inadequately met medical, housing, sanitation, education, and other basic needs.

Minority and disadvantaged groups lag behind the U.S. population on health status indicators (DHHS, 1990). For example, black

Americans, compared with the general population, have higher rates of high blood pressure, stroke, diabetes, and diseases associated with obesity (DHHS, 1988). Native Americans and Hispanics suffer greater disease and mortality burdens than whites (DHHS, 1985). Surveys indicate that people with the most education and other resources have made and benefited from dietary changes, whereas the poor and less educated have not (Heimbach, 1985). To lessen the burden of chronic disease and premature death for all its citizens, the nation will need to do more than implement recommendations on diet.[1] It also needs to be more accommodating to the diverse cultures of its people and focus its health promotion and outreach efforts on segments of the population that are least likely to eat well or practice other healthful behaviors.

BARRIERS AND INCENTIVES TO DIETARY CHANGE

Attempts to change dietary behavior are confronted with a particular set of problems. First, eating is often social and fun. Thus, many of the food choices that health-care professionals tend to view as undesirable are seen by the public as sources of pleasure. The committee does not wish to have people focus on health alone in deciding what to eat but, rather, to encourage them to modify their eating behaviors in ways that are both healthful and perceived as pleasurable. This is a challenging task.

Promotion of dietary change among healthy people may be an especially formidable problem for another reason: modifying eating behaviors, unlike quitting smoking, for example, usually produces few immediate physical or psychological benefits. Moreover, as Carmody and colleagues pointed out, people are being asked to move away from what "was and is the normal diet . . . for the U.S. population" rather than to abandon a recognizably pathogenic behavior (Carmody et al., 1986, p. 21).

Events that draw the public's attention to competing risks can be another barrier to dietary change. For example, at the time of release of the *Diet and Health* report, with its recommendations to consume fruits, vegetables, and poultry, the National Resources Defense Council warned that children were excessively exposed to agricultural chemicals, especially to Alar on apples (NRDC, 1989). Two weeks later, all fruit imported from Chile was temporarily barred from sale while the U.S. government sought to learn whether the cyanide discovered in two seedless grapes was widely dispersed among fruit distributed throughout the United States (Food Chemical News, 1989a). At about the same time, 400,000 chickens were destroyed in Arkansas because they were found to be contaminated with heptachlor, a cancer-causing pesticide that had been barred from agricultural use 11 years earlier (Food Chemical News, 1989b; Schneider, 1989).

Many health-care professionals see such alarms as a diversion of the public's attention away from more serious food-related issues. They argue that the hazard, if any, from chemical residues is much smaller than the known hazard of excessive fat consumption (NRC, 1989c). However, the evidence shows that the public is generally more concerned about a risk it cannot personally control (like pesticide residues) than one it can (like eating less fat) (NRC, 1989d). If health-care professionals want people to accept and follow their advice regarding health-promoting behaviors, they cannot afford to discount—or to view as distractions—the risks that most concern the public at any given moment.

Given the right incentives, people can surmount barriers to implementing dietary recommendations. For the individual, incentives to eat well include the likelihood that healthy dietary patterns—especially when combined with other behaviors—will enhance health and reduce the risk of many diseases. Furthermore, there are increasing opportunities today for consumers to select and prepare health-promoting and appealing meals that fit into their ways of life.[2] For the private sector, there are financial incentives to address the public's interest in better nutrition by developing more appealing food products with reduced levels of fat, sodium, and sugar. Because dietary improvements can be expected to improve the nation's health, governments and health-care professionals have a powerful reason to serve as role models and agenda setters for efforts to encourage more healthful food consumption practices and to coordinate, study, and monitor implementation efforts. These and other incentives to implement dietary recommendations are discussed in later chapters.

THE TASK OF IMPLEMENTATION: GOALS, TACTICS, AND POLICIES

Implementation begins with getting information about dietary recommendations to consumers in languages and formats that are relevant and comprehensible to them, given their diversities. The information provided must identify the components of a healthful diet and link such a diet to a life relatively freer of disease and disability.

The next and more difficult step is helping people to alter their food consumption practices in more healthful directions. This involves both individual and public responsibility. Society should not ignore the needs of people who have decided to move toward more healthful food consumption practices but find it difficult to do so. All sectors of society—including industry, government, and health-care professionals—have a responsibility to help individuals make and implement choices that result in the consumption of nutritionally desirable foods. To encourage better eating, health-promoting food choices must be accessible, easy to identify and prepare, economical, enjoyable, and adaptable to various life-styles. The committee's strategies and actions for implementation are designed to make it easier for people to eat healthful diets without sacrificing convenience or desired life-styles.

Implementation efforts must also take into account the so-called hidden choices that consumers rarely recognize and over which they have little or no control. These choices, which are made by others for consumers, include, for example, the ingredients used by restaurants (e.g., the types of fats and oils in which foods are cooked). Society has an obligation to ensure that such hidden choices are, whenever possible, made in a way that fosters healthful eating.

The goal of implementation efforts is to help people whose diets are less than ideal to reduce their intake of certain food components and increase their intake of others, i.e., to increase the prevalence of eating patterns that conform to dietary recommendations. This goal will be met in the following ways:

• enhancing awareness, understanding, and acceptance of dietary recommendations;
• creating legislative, regulatory, commercial, and educational environments supportive of the recommendations; and
• improving the availability of foods and meals that facilitate implementation of the recommendations.

The general tactics for increasing the prevalence of healthful eating patterns can be divided into three classes:

1. *Altering the food supply*—by *subtraction* (e.g., reducing the fat in meat and cheese), *addition* (e.g., appropriate fortification of foods with nutrients), and *substitution* (e.g., replacing some of the fat in margarine with water).

2. *Altering the food acquisition environment*—by providing *more food choices* that help consumers meet dietary recommendations, *better information* (e.g., more complete and interpretable product labeling), *advice at points of purchase* (e.g., tags indicating a good nutrition buy in supermarkets or cafeterias), and *more options* for selecting healthful diets (e.g, better food choices in vending machines and restaurants).

3. *Altering nutrition education*—by *changing the message mix* (e.g., presenting consistent messages in education programs, advertisements

for products, and public service announcements) and by *broadening exposure to formal and nonformal nutrition education* (e.g., mandating education on dietary recommendations from kindergarten through grade 12, in health-care facilities, and in medical schools).

Although common sense suggests that desirable dietary changes will most likely occur when all these components are made to be mutually reinforcing, there is insufficient research on their individual effectiveness or how they can best be assembled into a package. The attitudes and skills involved in carrying out these various kinds of interventions belong to different academic, institutional, sectoral, and societal domains; no substantial effort has been made until now to ask which combination of approaches offers the best promise of success in bringing about dietary change on a national level. In Chapter 3, the committee examines the evidence from community-based studies to learn which components of integrated programs of dietary change are associated with success.

THE TASK AND THE IMPLEMENTORS

In approaching the task of proposing strategies and actions for the nationwide implementation of dietary recommendations in the United States, the committee has taken a somewhat unconventional route. Rather than providing a simple list of all the steps that might be taken to modify diets, it has developed a list of interventions that seem most likely to work—given the need to protect free choice and to operate within resource limits. The committee has done this because it believes that consideration of implementation measures without regard to strongly held values and existing resource constraints is of little practical value. At the same time, it recognizes that conclusions regarding both values and resource constraints are subjective.

The committee began its work by imagining a wide range of strategies for modifying eating behavior. To the extent possible, each of these was examined in terms of such criteria as history of effectiveness, affordability, political feasibility, public acceptability, and legal and ethical considerations. Together, these criteria served as the basis for selecting implementation strategies and actions that in the committee's judgment are likely to be successful.

Much of the committee's work was done by four task forces, each focusing on specific societal sectors: public, private, health-care professions, and public education. These groupings were an effective mechanism for identifying the main interventions that have been attempted to date and for recommending those that might be undertaken in the future. The recommendations of these task forces are presented in Chapters 5 through 8.

It is clear that the four sectors have overlapping responsibilities. For example, all sectors use the media to inform and educate and to influence the public's diet-related behaviors. Governments make policies related to meat grading, to labeling, and to the kinds of foods offered in the school lunch and other food programs, thereby affecting the food supply, the shopping environment (private sector), and the educational environment. Mandates for nutrition education in the nation's classrooms from Congress or state legislatures obviously have the potential for changing the demands on health-care professionals as well.

There is a critical need for substantial government involvement and support in any comprehensive attempt to implement dietary recommendations. A key responsibility of governments is to serve as a role model and agenda setter. Public officials must ensure that all branches of government at all levels (federal, state, and local) work toward implementation of dietary recommendations by these steps: (1) initiate or expand practices that conform to dietary recommendations in dining facilities in government buildings; (2) reconcile legislation, regulations, policies, and practices so that they foster the effort; (3) use government's convening, educational, and technical assistance functions to urge private and voluntary groups to improve food selection and consumption patterns; and (4) capitalize on government's role in setting the diet and health agenda and its leadership in rallying and coordinating support.

Actions taken by the private sector are also cross-cutting. The producers, processors, and purveyors of food affect the food supply in many ways. For example, processors and marketers influence the food acquisition and educational environments through the information they provide on their packages and in their advertising messages and by the development and introduction of new food items that vary in their nutritional desirability. (An average of 34 new varieties of food and beverage products were introduced each day in the United States in 1989 [Shapiro, 1990].) Producer and processor groups directly influence classroom education through the creation and distribution of educational materials designed for use in schools. It is less apparent how much educators can affect the food supply or food acquisition environment, although they could hope to alter consumer demand and thus affect the actions of both the food industry and governments. These interrelationships speak to the need for collaboration and joint planning of implementation efforts.

All implementation efforts are constrained by the reality that no government or private or voluntary organization has the power to command the public to adopt a more healthful diet. Thus, the committee has also examined the issue of free choice as it relates to making informed food product choices while the number of choices continues to increase (see Chapter 8). Governments, industry, and voluntary health organizations lack financial resources, the ability to coordinate activities among them, and adequate staff and expertise to give technical assistance. At present, implementation is further constrained by insufficient knowledge—not so much of detailed relationships between diet and disease as of the environment in which change is being implemented. Too little is known about people's nutritional health because of the lack of comprehensive nutritional surveillance, and too little is known about the composition of the food supply and how that changes because of inadequate monitoring of these variables. Throughout its deliberations, the committee continually reminded itself of both resource and knowledge limitations and of the inevitable constraints on government effectiveness.

Chapter 9 contains the committee's directions for research. These are aimed at generating the knowledge that will improve the ability to design successful implementation strategies and actions.

BENEFITS AND COSTS OF DIETARY CHANGE

Public health programs are continually starved for resources. Thus, it is important that the resources available be used efficiently and that cost-effective projects, i.e., those that accomplish the goals at the lowest cost, receive first priority.

Devoting resources to implementing dietary recommendations is a public health project that must compete with other public health projects for resources. How much should be spent on media campaigns, improved labeling, or developing a manual to advise consumers on how to meet dietary recommendations? A careful assessment of the benefits and costs of each action and of the distribution of these benefits and costs is needed to make informed decisions about the allocation of resources.

Full implementation of dietary recommendations promises considerable benefits in improved health and well-being and fewer costs for work absence and disability. Unfortunately, implemention of dietary recommendations will sometimes be difficult and costly. The costs include (1) the monetary costs of establishing and maintaining the programs and structures that educate consumers about dietary recommendations and how to implement them; (2) the costs incurred by the private sector in changing production, manufacturing, and processing practices to emphasize foods that help people to meet dietary recommendations; and (3) the psychological costs that some people will bear by taking up a new diet that is perceived to be less satisfying and more troublesome to buy and prepare—at least in the short run. Because implementation of almost any of the recommendations in this report will have effects that go well beyond nutritional ones, it is important that hidden costs and benefits be identified beforehand, to the extent possible. For example, committee recommendations to modify the formulation of certain foods might raise the price of these products, at least in the short term—a hidden cost.

Given the time and resource constraints for this study, the benefits and costs of the proposed actions could not be estimated with confidence. The primary difficulty is the lack of quantification of the effects of past programs to modify dietary practices or observe the health effects of dietary modifications. The committee recommends strongly that the plan for every action undertaken to modify dietary habits include adequate evaluation, which will require adequate resources. Such evaluations would indicate which programs should be expanded, which ones should be modified (and when the modification is successful), and which ones should be discontinued as unsuccessful.

NOTES

1. Several reports from the National Research Council and Institute of Medicine address the medical, social, and public welfare needs of the poor in the United States. These reports include: *Risking the Future: Adolescent Sexuality, Pregnancy, and Childbearing* (NRC, 1987), *Prenatal Care: Reaching Mothers, Reaching Infants* (IOM, 1988b), *Homelessness, Health, and Human Needs* (IOM, 1988a), *Who Cares for America's Children?* (NRC, 1990), *A Common Destiny: Blacks and American Society* (NRC, 1989b), *AIDS, Sexual Behavior, and Intravenous Drug Use* (NRC, 1989a), *Confronting AIDS: Update 1988* (IOM, 1989), *Broadening the Base of Treatment for Alcohol Problems* (IOM, 1990), and *Alcohol in America: Taking Action to Prevent Abuse* (NRC, 1985). A recent report by the Life Sciences Research Office addresses nutrition problems among disadvantaged, difficult-to-sample populations (LSRO, 1990).

2. Health-care professionals are in general agreement that all foods that contribute to healthful diets are, by definition, health promoting and that any food that supplies energy and nutrients can be nutritionally desirable. There is also general agreement that dietary recommendations should not prohibit the consumption of any food product and that the nutritional composition of the total diet is of more importance than is that of a single food or meal. However, for practical purposes, the committee uses the terms *health promoting* and *nutritionally desirable* to describe foods whose consumption is encouraged to meet dietary recommendations. Examples include fruits, vegetables, and breads. In addition, the committee describes a *healthful* diet as one that meets dietary recommendations most of the time (and is thereby composed largely of health-promoting foods) and that meets nutrient needs.

REFERENCES

Carmody, T.P., J. Istvan, J.D. Matarazzo, S.L. Connor, and W.E. Connor. 1986. Applications of social learning theory in the promotion of heart-healthy diets: the Family Heart Study dietary intervention model. Health Educ. Res. 1:13-27.

DHEW (U.S. Department of Health, Education, and Welfare). 1979. Healthy People: the Surgeon General's Report on Health Promotion and Disease Prevention. DHEW (PHS) Publ. No. 79-55071. Office of the Assistant Secretary for Health and Surgeon General, Public Health Service, U.S. Department of Health, Education, and Welfare. U.S. Government Printing Office, Washington, D.C. 177 pp.

DHHS (U.S. Department of Health and Human Services). 1980. Promoting Health/ Preventing Disease: Objectives for the Nation. Public Health Service, U.S. Department of Health and Human Services. U.S. Government Printing Office, Washington, D.C. 102 pp.

DHHS (U.S. Department of Health and Human Services). 1985. Report of the Secretary's Task Force on Black & Minority Health. Volume II: Crosscutting Issues in Minority Health. U.S. Department of Health and Human Services, Washington, D.C. 549 pp.

DHHS (U.S. Department of Health and Human Services). 1988. The Surgeon General's Report on Nutrition and Health. DHHS (PHS) Publ. No. 88-50210. Public Health Service, U.S. Department of Health and Human Services. U.S. Government Printing Office, Washington, D.C. 727 pp.

DHHS (U.S. Department of Health and Human Services). 1990. Healthy People 2000: National Health Promotion and Disease Prevention Objectives. Conference edition. Public Health Service, U.S. Department of Health and Human Services. U.S. Government Printing Office, Washington, D.C. 672 pp.

FMI (Food Marketing Institute). 1990. Trends: Consumer Attitudes & the Supermarket, 1990. Conducted for Food Marketing Institute by Opinion Research Corporation. The Research Department, Food Marketing Institute, Washington, D.C. 70 pp.

Food Chemical News. 1989a. FDA announces Class II nationwide recall of Chilean fruit. Food Chem. News 31(6):36-38.

Food Chemical News. 1989b. State to warn customers of heptachlor-contaminated feed. Food Chem. News 31(6):42.

Haughton, B., J.D. Gussow, and J.M. Dodds. 1987. An historical study of the underlying assumptions for United States food guides from 1917 through the Basic Four Food Group Guide. J. Nutr. Educ. 19:169-176.

Heimbach, J.T. 1985. Cardiovascular disease and diet: the public view. Public Health Rep. 100:5-12.

IOM (Institute of Medicine). 1988a. Homelessness, Health, and Human Needs. Report of the Committee on Health Care for Homeless People. National Academy Press, Washington, D.C. 242 pp.

IOM (Institute of Medicine). 1988b. Prenatal Care: Reaching Mothers, Reaching Infants. Report of the Committee to Study Outreach for Prenatal Care, Division of Health Promotion and Disease Prevention. National Academy Press, Washington, D.C. 254 pp.

IOM (Institute of Medicine). 1989. Confronting AIDS: Update 1988. Report of the Committee for the Oversight of AIDS Activities. National Academy Press, Washington, D.C. 239 pp.

IOM (Institute of Medicine). 1990. Broadening the Base of Treatment for Alcohol Problems: Report of a Study. Report of the Committee for the Study of Treatment and Rehabilitation Services for Alcoholism and Alcohol Problems, Division of Men-

tal Health and Behavioral Medicine. National Academy Press, Washington, D.C. 900 pp.
LSRO (Life Sciences Research Office). 1990. Core Indicators of Nutritional State for Difficult-to-Sample Populations. Federation of American Societies for Experimental Biology, Bethesda, Md. 63 pp.
Mayer, J. 1990. Hunger and undernutrition in the United States. J. Nutr. 120:919-923.
NCEP (National Cholesterol Education Program). 1990. Report of the Expert Panel on Population Strategies for Blood Cholesterol Reduction. NIH Publication No. 90-3046. National Heart, Lung, and Blood Institute, National Institutes of Health, U.S. Department of Health and Human Services. 139 pp.
NRC (National Research Council). 1985. Alcohol in America: Taking Action to Prevent Abuse. Report of the Panel on Alternative Policies Affecting the Prevention of Alcohol Abuse and Alcoholism, Commission on Behavioral and Social Sciences and Education. National Academy Press, Washington, D.C. 125 pp.
NRC (National Research Council). 1987. Risking the Future: Adolescent Sexuality, Pregnancy, and Childbearing. Report of the Panel on Adolescent Pregnancy and Childbearing, Committee on Child Development Research and Public Policy, Commission on Behavioral and Social Sciences and Education. National Academy Press, Washington, D.C. 337 pp.
NRC (National Research Council). 1989a. AIDS, Sexual Behavior, and Intravenous Drug Use. Report of the Committee on AIDS Research and the Behavioral, Social, and Statistical Sciences, Commission on Behavioral and Social Sciences and Education. National Academy Press, Washington, D.C. 589 pp.
NRC (National Research Council). 1989b. A Common Destiny: Blacks and American Society. Report of the Committee on the Status of Black Americans, Commission on Behavioral and Social Sciences and Education. National Academy Press, Washington, D.C. 624 pp.
NRC (National Research Council). 1989c. Diet and Health: Implications for Reducing Chronic Disease Risk. Report of the Committee on Diet and Health, Food and Nutrition Board, Commission on Life Sciences. National Academy Press, Washington, D.C. 749 pp.
NRC (National Research Council). 1989d. Improving Risk Communication. Report of the Committee on Risk Perception and Communication, Commission on Behavioral and Social Sciences and Education, Commission on Physical Sciences, Mathematics, and Resources. National Academy Press, Washington, D.C. 332 pp.
NRC (National Research Council). 1990. Who Cares for America's Children? Child Care Policy for the 1990s. Report of the Panel on Child Care Policy, Commission on Behavioral and Social Sciences and Education. National Academy Press, Washington, D.C. 347 pp.
NRDC (National Resources Defense Council). 1989. Intolerable Risk: Pesticides in Our Children's Food. National Resources Defense Council, Washington, D.C. 141 pp.
Schneider, K. March 16, 1989. Pesticide barred in 70's is found to taint poultry. New York Times. A16.
Shapiro, E. May 29, 1990. New products clog foodstores. New York Times. D1, D17.
Stoto, M.A., R. Behrens, and C. Rosemont, eds. 1990. Healthy People 2000: Citizens Chart the Course. National Academy Press, Washington, D.C. 228 pp.
U.S. Congress, Senate. 1909. Report of the President's Homes Commission. Committee on District of Columbia. U.S. Senate Document No. 644, 60th Congress, 2nd session. U.S. Government Printing Office, Washington, D.C. 159 pp.
U.S. Congress, Senate. 1977a. Dietary Goals for the United States. Report of the Select

Committee on Nutrition and Human Needs. Stock No. 052-070-03913-2. U.S. Government Printing Office, Washington, D.C. 79 pp.

U.S. Congress, Senate. 1977b. Dietary Goals for the United States, 2nd ed. Report of the Select Committee on Nutrition and Human Needs. Stock No. 052-070-04376-8. U.S. Government Printing Office, Washington, D.C. 83 pp.

USDA (U.S. Department of Agriculture). 1989. Preparing Foods & Planning Menus Using Dietary Guidelines. Home and Garden Bulletin No. 232-8. Human Nutrition Information Service, U.S. Department of Agriculture, Hyattsville, Md. 32 pp.

USDA/DHHS (U.S. Department of Agriculture/U.S. Department of Health and Human Services). 1980. Nutrition and Your Health: Dietary Guidelines for Americans. Home and Garden Bulletin No. 228. U.S. Department of Agriculture and U.S. Department of Health and Human Services, Washington, D.C. 20 pp.

USDA/DHHS (U.S. Department of Agriculture/U.S. Department of Health and Human Services). 1990. Nutrition and Your Health: Dietary Guidelines for Americans, 3rd ed. Home and Garden Bulletin No. 232. U.S. Department of Agriculture and U.S. Department of Health and Human Services, Washington, D.C. 28 pp.

3
Determinants of Food Choice and Prospects for Modifying Food Attitudes and Behavior

M ANY CHANGES have taken place in the United States during the past century with respect to food selection and attitudes toward diet and health. In this chapter, these changes are reviewed by the committee as are the prospects for future changes in behaviors and attitudes to meet dietary recommendations. The focus is on the general U.S. population rather than specific high-risk groups.

Recommendations for changing eating habits are more likely to be adopted if their framers (1) are knowledgeable about the factors known to affect food choices, (2) recognize current trends in food consumption and attitudes toward food, (3) base their recommendations on basic theory and research related to changing attitudes and behaviors, and (4) learn from previous attempts to change diet for health purposes. This chapter is organized to address each of these items in sequence. To select the most appropriate targets of change (e.g., the most critical beliefs or behaviors), one must know the basic determinants of food choice and which of these are subject to modification. Likewise, it would not be prudent to recommend specific methods or programs of change without knowledge of basic theory and research on the determinants of behavior change and of the techniques that have already proven successful. For example, it is critical to understand why an individual's knowledge alone about the links between diet and health is unlikely to change dietary behavior. It is also important to know what changes are already taking place in the United States and whether these trends are likely to facilitate or hinder implementation of dietary recommendations.

33

This chapter concludes with a critical review of some intervention programs designed explicitly to improve eating patterns. These include programs instituted at the individual, organizational, and community levels.

DETERMINANTS OF FOOD CHOICE

Why any group of humans eats what it does is considerably more difficult to explain than is the eating behavior of other species. In humans, appetite is not simply a physiological drive toward food but, rather, a complex set of physical, emotional, and cognitive stimuli compounded from events widely separated in time and space.

Because humans from birth through childhood depend for their survival on nurturance provided by other members of their species, they are uniquely vulnerable to developing affective relationships with food and feeders. Thus, nourishment for humans almost inevitably becomes associated with powerful emotional attachments. These, overlaid with beliefs and feelings that continue to accumulate around food consumption as individuals mature, combine with immediate environmental stimuli to direct food choices.

Beneath their socialization, however, humans remain animals, endowed with sets of sensors that underlie all their subsequent encounters with food. Taste is one of these. The evidence is overwhelming, for example, that humans are innately programmed to like sweet tastes at birth—and even in utero (Montagu, 1962; Weiffenbach, 1977), and there are very tentative indications that they are also born with some sort of attraction to meat, to its fat, or to both (Beauchamp and Moran, 1982; Drewnowski et al., 1985; Farb and Armelagos, 1980; Harris, 1985). Since many poisons are bitter and fruits become sweeter as they ripen toward greater nutritiousness, a taste for sweetness may well have given its possessor a selective advantage. A preference for fat would also have favored survival under conditions of calorie deprivation.

Humans also like salt, although it is not an innately preferred taste in infancy (Davis, 1928; Steiner, 1977). People who change to low-salt foods come to consider formerly acceptable foods too salty. Thus, the preferred level of saltiness appears to be strongly affected by experience. Such is not the case for sweetness, however; preferences for different levels of sweetness appear to be inborn (Desor et al., 1977). The ability to taste certain isolated flavor chemicals (e.g., phenylthiocarbamide) varies with individuals and is genetically controlled. Although there appears to be little genetic control over the liking for particular foods (Fabsitz et al., 1980), early research on food choice suggested that infants protected from poisonous foods and exposed only to uncombined foods whose indigenous components have been neither concentrated nor diluted with added fat, salt, or sweeteners are able to select fully nutritious diets instinctively (Davis, 1928). Humans also appear to be born with automatic regulators of energy need (of a complexity not yet deciphered) that are set differently at or before birth (Ravussin et al., 1988; Roberts et al., 1988).

This physiological base on which eating behavior is built appears to explain very little about the food choices people actually make. The experiences of individuals as members of specific families in a particular culture tend almost inevitably to overwhelm many (if not all) the signals coming from what Jean Mayer long ago called the "animal within" (Mayer, 1968). Young babies universally find chili aversive. Yet, as Rozin and Schiller (1980) have demonstrated, this innate aversion to chili, along with the innate preference for sweets, is spontaneously overcome in Mexican children, almost half of whom at age 6 or 7 years will select a spicy hot snack over a sweet one when given a choice. In an earlier classic study, Moskowitz et al. (1975) found that chronic exposure to tamarind among a group of Asian Indians overrode the relative dislike of the sour taste characteristic among humans. As indicated by the prevalence of overweight people in the United States, culture can also override in humans the bodyweight-regulating mechanism that operates effectively in all other species (except when they are domesticated).

Factors other than physiological ones that affect food choice can all be attributed to either nurture or culture. However, since culture heavily affects the ways in which a society nurtures, even this division is somewhat artificial. One such factor is early feeding experiences, which involve, in addition to tastes and smells, the sounds, sights, textures, and emotions associated with feeders. Thus, they deeply affect infants who are entirely dependent on their feeders for survival. These individual feelings about eating, implanted in infancy, may be difficult to modify. There is evidence that food aversions resulting from even a single, powerful negative experience with a food can be very long lasting (Garb and Stunkard, 1974). Therefore, if patterns established in early infancy need modification, recommendations would need to be directed to food providers, usually parents.

There is no direct evidence, however, that food preferences learned in infancy are permanent, but there has been little systematic study of early feeding interactions and their effects on later eating behaviors. "There are currently no prospective or longitudinal data with human subjects to provide support for [the] assumption that early food acceptance patterns are . . . reflected in food acceptance patterns later in life" (Birch, 1987, p. 127). Nor is it known what makes certain children like certain foods. Davis (1928) found that infants previously unexposed to any food but mother's milk, and protected from outside influences on food choice, expressed a wide range of preferences when they were allowed to choose from a variety of simply prepared, unsalted, unsweetened foods. Birch (1987), who investigated food acceptance by young children, concluded that "sweetness" and "familiarity" were two characteristics of food that seemed largely to account for children's food choices in the United States. In this country, preschoolers are almost unavoidably often exposed to highly sweetened foods; thus, the sweetness factor that drives food acceptability in this and similar cultures may arise in large part from familiarity, as may the preference for spicy hot foods in Mexico. There is evidence that continuous exposure to sweetness sustains the neonate's preference for sweetness (Beauchamp and Moran, 1982).

Davis (1934) could not determine whether the initial food choices of infants in her study were random or whether they were based on color, odor, or both. It is known that children's acceptance of food can be influenced by the choices of their eating companions (Birch, 1987). Since parents or other caretakers normally select the foods to be made available to very young children and their eating companions, adults have a strong influence over children's food choices. In the United States, however, children are exposed from early infancy to adults other than members of their own households who tell them what to eat. Many of these adults are seen on television, advertising edible products consisting largely of sugared cereals, candy, and fast-service foods. A recent study in Québec indicated that the parents of children who watch child-oriented television that carries commercials purchase more brands of breakfast cereal directed specifically toward children than do the parents of children who watch commercial-free children's programming (Goldberg and Hartwick, 1990). Thus, advertising demonstrably influences parents as they select food products for their children.

In a study of influences on the food choices of elementary school children and adolescents, Contento and Michela found the two most important variables in both groups to be "parents serve it" and "tastes good" (Contento et al., 1988; Michela and Contento, 1986). Taste predominated among the adolescents; serving by parents took first place among the younger children. Although the sweetness variable was not examined directly in either study, the same authors found in an earlier investigation that sweetness was a highly salient dimension in children's spontaneous classification of foods into groups (Michela and Contento, 1984).

Examining adolescent food choices more closely, Contento et al. (1988) found that their subjects could be divided into subgroups "with different motivations for food choice—irrespective of ethnicity and gender" (p. 297). Subjects at one extreme were "hedonistic"—choosing foods even if they could identify those foods as causing heart disease or containing sugar or fat. Subjects at the other extreme were "health oriented" in that they avoided these same foods and ate foods they perceived as "healthful." Although the food choices of peers were reported to be an important influence on the "hedonistic" group and on others, it was not an important factor in all subgroups. The evidence thus suggests that children, some of them even into adolescence, are heavily influenced by their parents' choices of food to serve. As they grow older, however, some children choose foods they perceive as healthful or unhealthful; others are more strongly influenced by other social and environmental factors and by taste.

Many of the factors known to affect food choice beyond adolescence cannot readily be modified by educational or other populationwide interventions. These include individuals' positive or aversive food or eating experiences that may make certain foods especially palatable or nauseatingly unacceptable, as well as simple familiarity, which probably plays an important role in determining food choice in adulthood just as it does among children. But even though education cannot change an individual's historic relationship with certain foods, food likes and dislikes can be modified with further experience; a new and wholesome food, once tried, may become both familiar and liked.

Other variables often identified as determining food choices in adults include age, sex, race, place of birth, time of day, season of year, marital status, children's ages, household size, employment status, income, and—perhaps less obviously—media events affecting the public's perception of the safety or wholesomeness of the food supply. Although none of these determinants of food selection can be intentionally altered by policymakers, many of them can change over relatively short or long periods. For example, women's increasing participation in the work force encourages more frequent eating outside the home. People at different ages or at different stages of their life cycles will also respond differently to messages about food. For example, the population as a whole is aging (DHHS, 1988), and an aging population is likely to be more aware of and concerned about health and may therefore be more disposed to seek out certain food components (e.g., fiber and calcium) or avoid others (e.g., fat).

Much of the research concerned with modifiable determinants of food selection has been conducted either by marketers attempting to determine which appeals will be most effective in selling products or by researchers interested in the factors that promote overeating. Yankelovich, Skelly and White, Inc. (1985) identified "convenience," "price," "nutrition," "variety," "quality," and "good taste" as the variables that will establish "competitive parameters for those who will serve tomorrow's consumers." Rodin (1980), listing "social and immediate environmental influences on food selection," identified "time of day," "accessibility/availability," "expedience," "variety," "media effects," "conditioned stimuli," and "emotions."

Many of the factors on both lists are not directly relevant to the question in this chapter: what factors can be manipulated to affect food choice in a healthful direction? The only common factor on the lists is *variety*, which often represents to a marketer a way of getting a larger share of the market. In that sense, variety is related to *newness*, which appears to be an inducement to consumers to at least try a product. Evidence indicates that a monotonous diet leads to decreased food consumption and the availability of a variety of tasty foods leads to increased calorie intake, even among animals who are normally very good at self-regulation (Sclafani and Springer, 1976). Humans may have room for a dessert even when they are entirely satiated from previous courses. Thus, increased variety is unlikely to be helpful in a situation where overconsumption is part of the problem.

Price is often mentioned as influencing food choice, and it has played an important role in at least two major health-related dietary changes: the shift from butter to margarine that began during World War II (Green, 1975) and the shift from red meat to chicken that began in earnest in 1976. Between 1976 and 1987, chicken consumption increased by 48% while the average retail price of chicken as a percentage of the price of beef decreased from 40 to 32% (Putnam, 1989). The importance of price as a factor affecting food choice obviously varies, however, with the proportion of the family budget spent on food. Although increased income does not necessarily lead to an improvement in dietary quality, inadequate funds may limit consumption of costly fish and (at certain seasons) certain fresh fruits and vegetables. Many other health-promoting foods (e.g., breads and other grain products, starchy tubers, and dry beans) are relatively cheap, and many less desirable foods (e.g., sweet and salty snacks, rich desserts, and heavily marbled beef) are relatively expensive. Thus, price, combined with appropriate education, is a variable that could in some cases favor adoption of dietary recommendations.

Very little is known about how individuals (or populations) acquire taste preferences. Familiarity appears to be important among adults as well as among children; however, what tastes good or appropriate at a given time to any one person undoubtedly relates to some of the factors identified by Rodin (1980), for example, "conditioned stimuli" (a cocktail with the evening news, popcorn at the movies, hot cocoa at bedtime), "emotions" (candy during times of sadness), or "time of day" (ham and eggs for breakfast). Food preferences governed by such factors would be amenable to change if education leads to changed social norms.

In discussing factors that affect food choice, a distinction must be made between what *is* and what is *perceived to be* reality by the potential consumer. In that sense, quality (like nutritiousness or healthfulness) is a belief factor. Quality can mean very different things to different consumers—all the way from the fact that a food bears a well-known brand name to the fact that it bears no brand name at all and is purchased fresh from the farmer who produced it. The characteristics of foods that groups of people associate with quality can obviously change over time (e.g., among certain groups, marbling in beef has been replaced as a quality factor by beef raised without hormones).

Nutritiousness has recently become identifiable as one characteristic of a quality product, although no more than 15 years ago, manufacturers resisted nutritional marketing appeals on the grounds that people were simply not interested (Belasco, 1989). At present, consumers will, at least some of the time, select food they *believe* to be nutritious. Perceived nutritiousness, especially in a food already highly desired, is a selling tool.

Low calorie is another quality appeal in a culture in which at any given time 33% of women and a smaller percentage of men claim to be dieting (Calorie Control Council, 1989). The astonishing success of the marketing of diet soft drinks, whose consumption shot up from approximately 1 to 8 gallons per capita between 1954 and 1987 (USDA, 1989), is a clear indicator that identifying a product as *diet* or *low calorie* will increase the likelihood that it will be selected by a substantial segment of the population. The selling of the potato as a low-calorie food (Dugas, 1985; Ketchum Communications, 1989) is an example of a marketing approach that might be used to some advantage in implementing dietary recommendations.

The fact that $3.7 billion is spent annually on food advertising (Advertising Age, 1989) has led to a popular conviction that advertising, especially on television, is a major influence on food choice. Although advertising agencies survive by convincing clients that this is true, the direct effects of the media on food selection are difficult to isolate from all the other promotional factors to which an individual is exposed. Advertising induces people to try new products that might otherwise go unnoticed; it has encouraged the belief that all thirst must be quenched from a bottle—not from the water tap; it can lead consumers to switch from one brand of soda or tuna to another; and the repeated picturing on television of highly palatable food may induce snacking (Falciglia and Gussow, 1980).

Of all the factors affecting food selection, two—availability of foods and knowledge of and beliefs about foods and health—are perhaps the most powerful of those amenable to modification. Availability is a much less obvious concept than it seems, incorporating such notions as convenience and technological progress.

Real availability—the presence of enough varied food to eat—is not an issue in the United States, where variety and quantity abound. However, the sheer number of choices does sometimes constrain availability, since food stores tend to feature the products that sell fastest, so that, for example, refined flour products have been more readily available than those made of whole grains. Nevertheless, certain desirable products such as lower-fat meat and a greater variety of fresh fruits and vegetables are now becoming increasingly available (Duewer, 1989; Greene, 1988).

Perceived availability is a different sort of factor. It changes over time among different groups with different skills and expectations. For many people, a food is now considered to be available only when it can be acquired in a few minutes or is ready to eat at any time of the day or night at a nearby location. This definition of availability restricts many people's food choices; for example, what is available for immediate consumption in many settings may be limited to a variety of bottled liquids and a collection of small packaged snacks. Increasingly, especially in urban areas, there are specialty shops that sell foods with highly concentrated energy components—premium ice cream and freshly baked cookies, for example. With regard to these prepacked or preportioned street foods, it is usually more "expedient" (to use Rodin's word) to eat the whole thing—the whole cookie (however enormous), the whole package of crackers or nuts, or the whole bottle of beer or soda—regardless of actual appetite, since that is what is available. Because snacks and fast-service foods of all kinds are ubiquitous, they are seen as choices, even though they provide a limited variety and less control over fat, sodium, and sugar intake than people might want.

Convenience—a term applied to something that promises to save work or time—is a subset of availability. To someone who feels time-constrained, a food that requires extended preparation is not perceived as available. To someone without cooking skills, a raw chicken is not available. Technology's impact on food choices results partly from its ability to continually redefine perceived availability.

Microwave ovens, for example, lead to increased availability, and thus consumption, of microwavable snacks (Erickson, 1989). Thus, instant heating makes hot snack foods more available.

Cultural availability is important, because one's culture determines what constitutes food; all cultures reject some edible parts of their environments. In the United States, dogs, cats, and horses are seldom eaten, although they are readily available, and Americans do not think of hunting birds and squirrels in parks. In many cultures, milk is considered to be an inappropriate food for adults, and in many others, bread is not spread with butter or margarine as it is in the United States. Because this country is relatively young and culturally diverse, it has no traditional national cuisine—no foods that most of its citizens have eaten for generations. Regional foods (e.g., baked beans and brown bread or grits and red-eye gravy) have tended to be displaced by the cuisine offered at franchise restaurants. This lack of a long-standing, strong food tradition may prove to be an advantage to those attempting to produce dietary changes directed toward health.

Cultural factors determine not only what but also when, where, how much, and how quickly food is to be eaten. Since the U.S. population has traditionally bolted its food (Fletcher, 1899), fast-service food is nothing really new. People in the United States also spend more time alone than people in many other countries do (Szalai, 1972) and they often eat alone—in cars, at their desks, by the refrigerator, or close to vending machines (Lantis, 1962). Foods are increasingly available in quantities designed to be eaten alone, which means that any attempt to alter eating patterns must be directed at different population segments, not merely at adults, since they are no longer the "gatekeepers" identified by Lewin (1943). Efforts to affect eating patterns need to be attentive to these ambiguous cultural messages since *what* will be eaten is so often dependent on where, when, and how quickly it is to be eaten.

As documented later in this chapter, consumers have become more concerned about the relationship between diet and health and report that they are trying to change their diets accordingly. This interest is confirmed by the increasing emphasis on healthfulness as an important food marketing tool. During the past few decades, there have been substantial changes in overall food consumption patterns (Putnam, 1989). Survey data show a widespread *verbal* commitment to eating for health, but consumption data show that declining consumption of beef, eggs, butter, whole milk, and other traditional contributors of saturated fat and cholesterol has been countered somewhat by a rising consumption of cheese, premium ice cream, and other rich sources of saturated fat (Popkin et al., 1989; Putnam, 1989). In providing consumers with information that will allow or induce them to act on their stated health concerns, attention will need to be paid to helping them place the confusing bits of information they encounter into a coherent overall picture of the association of diet with health.

CHANGES IN FOOD SELECTION

It is evident from the preceding discussion that learning why people eat what they do is a complicated undertaking. Finding out exactly what individuals eat is only marginally easier (see, for example, NRC, 1989 and Woteki, 1986). It is possible, however, to obtain reasonably good data on overall changes in the U.S. food supply over time. These are useful for tracking trends in food demand and can be examined to learn whether food consumption patterns are changing in a direction consistent with dietary recommendations.

Changes in foods available to the public from 1909 to the present can be identified by examining U.S. Department of Agriculture (USDA) data on the disappearance of foods into wholesale and retail markets. The amounts of foods available to the public in a given year are estimated by subtracting data on exports, year-end inventories, and nonfood uses from data on total production, imports, and inventories at the beginning of the year. These quantities are larger than those actually consumed, since they do not include losses from processing, marketing, and home use (NRC, 1989; Putnam, 1989). USDA has also surveyed food use of households and dietary intakes and patterns of individuals in the Nationwide Food Consumption Surveys (NFCS) and the Continuing Surveys of Food Intake by Individuals (CSFII). Since the overall pattern of changes in both the NFCS and CSFII are generally consistent with the patterns shown in the disappearance data (Popkin et al., 1989), only the latter are presented here.

Table 3-1 presents the quantities of food available for consumption per person from periods extending from 1909 to 1987 (the latest data available when this report was prepared). Since data on some foods, especially processed vegetables and fruits, were not collected in the earlier years, comparisons of the consumption of these products over time are difficult to make.

Changes from 1909 to 1987

Since the first settlers arrived in a New World that was teeming with game, meat has had a dominant position in the diets of its inhabitants. Although beef consumption in 1987 was the lowest since the 1960s, it remained approximately 40 to 50% higher than that during World War II and the preceding years back to 1909. Much of the apparent decrease noted in 1987 may be misleading, however, since retail cuts were much more closely trimmed of fat in that year than they were in the past (Putnam, 1989). Thus, past disappearance data probably included some weight that was trimmed before consumption. Although year-to-year fluctuations in pork consumption have often been quite high, the long-term average weight of pork available per person has varied little during the past eight decades. The most remarkable change has occurred in poultry consumption, which now averages 78 lb per person—nearly five times higher than pre-World War II levels. This increased intake of poultry and a much smaller increase in fish consumption have more than made up for the decrease in beef, veal, and lamb. The annual consumption of total red meat, poultry, and fish in 1987 was not only the highest ever in the United States but it also exceeded that of the traditional leaders—Australia and New Zealand. Consumption of dairy products peaked in 1945. Per-capita consumption decreased until the 1960s and 1970s, when consumption of low-fat milk, cheese, and frozen dairy products such as ice cream began to increase. Low-fat milk (1 to 2% fat, skim, buttermilk, and some flavored milk) consumption almost doubled between 1971 and 1987, when consumption of low-fat milk overtook that of whole milk.

Egg consumption has decreased to 67% of its World War II high, but is only 15% less than its prewar level and has remained fairly constant in the 1980s. Although butter and margarine use combined has changed relatively little since the 1940s, margarine use has increased at the expense of butter. Consumption of fats and oils has steadily increased, reaching a point in 1987 that was approximately 50% higher than that recorded in the period from 1909 to 1913. Per-capita use of salad and cooking oils has increased markedly in the past two decades.

Data on average vegetable consumption are less clear than those for other food groups because the sources of these data have changed. For example, current data are no longer available on several vegetables. Putnam (1989) reported, however, that per-capita consumption of nine major fresh vegetables—asparagus, broccoli, carrots, cauliflower, celery, corn, lettuce, onions, and tomatoes—reached a record high in 1987. In the past decade, per-capita consumption of frozen vegetables has increased while consumption of canned vegetables has decreased. Based on disappearance data, fresh fruit consumption has increased dramatically in the past two decades. However, food consumption survey data give a somewhat different picture. According to USDA, consumption of fruits and vegetables among women ages 19 to 50 actually declined by an average of 7% between

TABLE 3-1 Quantities of Food Available for Consumption in the U.S. Food Supply^a

Item	Quantity Available for Per-Capita Consumption, lb^b					
	1909-1913	1929-1933	1944-1948	1970-1974	1975-1979	1987
Total red meat, poultry, and fish	153.8	139.0	159.5	211.8	214.7	277.1
Red meat^c	126.6	113.5	127.3	150.6	147.9	133.9
Beef	53.2	38.2	48.2	83.9	87.8	73.4
Veal	6.3	5.9	9.8	2.0	2.8	1.5
Pork	60.9	63.6	63.9	62.1	55.8	59.2
Lamb and mutton	6.2	5.8	5.4	2.6	1.5	1.3
Poultry	16.0	16.0	22.4	49.1	53.9	77.8
Chicken	14.9	14.4	19.3	40.5	44.8	62.7
Turkey	1.1	1.6	3.1	8.6	9.1	15.1
Fish^d	11.2	9.5	9.8	12.1	12.9	15.4
Fresh and frozen		5.2	6.0	7.0	7.9	10.0
Canned and cured		4.3	3.8	5.1	5.0	5.4
Eggs	36.8	38.5	46.5	37.9	34.6	31.6
Dairy products						
Fluid whole milk	265.0	270.2	317.4	205.2	168.4	109.9
Fluid low-fat milk	86.4	66.0	59.8	59.1	81.2	113.6
Cheese^e	4.0	4.5	6.3	12.9	16.0	24.0
Frozen dairy products	1.2	4.4	12.0	28.1	27.5	29.1
Fats and oils						
Butter	17.3	17.7	10.7	5.0	4.4	4.6
Margarine	1.3	2.1	4.5	11.0	11.4	10.5
Shortening	8.3	8.7	9.3	17.1	17.7	21.3
Lard and edible tallow	11.6	13.3	12.1	3.8	2.6	2.8
Salad and cooking oils	1.5	5.3	6.6	16.7	19.5	25.2

Fruit						
Fresh fruit	129.7	125.7	131.4	76.0	80.8	98.7
Citrus	13.5	35.4	58.1	27.2	26.4	27.2
Noncitrus	116.2	90.3	73.3	48.8	54.4	71.5
Processed fruit and juice				56.1	61.9	62.3
Vegetables						
Fresh vegetables, except potatoes	53.4	83.0	99.2	92.4	97.2	78.6[f]
Fresh potatoes	167.0	127.0	112.5	54.0	49.0	45.1
Processed vegetables, except potatoes				106.3	105.1	104.2
Processed potatoes				21.8	27.2	24.3
Grain products						
Wheat flour and cereal products	287.0	222.6	183.2	141.2	148.9	169.3
Wheat flour	210.0	168.0	147.0	111.0	116.3	128.0
Corn flour and meal	49.0	23.0	16.0	6.3	5.9	6.7
Pasta	NA[g]	NA	NA	8.5	10.1	17.1
Breakfast cereals	NA	NA	NA	11.0	12.6	15.2
Rice	7.0	5.6	4.7	7.1	7.5	13.4
Sweeteners						
Refined sugar	75.7	97.7	84.2	100.5	91.5	62.4
Syrup and corn sweeteners[h]	14.2	18.0	21.6	23.3	33.1	70.2

[a] SOURCES: Putnam (1989) and USDA (1953).
[b] Retail-weight equivalent. Based on total U.S. population and, except for 1944 to 1948, includes consumption by U.S. Armed Forces stationed overseas. Fluid milk consumption is based on U.S. resident (civilian and military) population, and fish consumption based on U.S. civilian population.
[c] Excludes consumption of game and edible offals.
[d] Edible weight.
[e] Product weight, excludes cottage cheese.
[f] Data for 1987 do not include artichokes, cabbage, cucumbers, eggplant, escarole, garlic, green beans, green peppers, spinach, and minor vegetables due to reporting cutbacks. Comparable figures for 1970-74 and 1975-79 are 65.0 and 68.4 lb, respectively.
[g] NA–Not Available.
[h] Corn sweeteners included only after 1969.

1977 and 1985 (USDA, 1985). The decline was most pronounced among low-income women (15% for fruits and 21% for vegetables).

Consumption of flour and grains has increased in recent years, following a dramatic drop during the first part of this century (Putnam, 1989). Average consumption of white flour has increased 15% in the past two decades, largely as a result of the greater demand for pasta. Breakfast cereal consumption was also up from 11 lb per capita in 1970 to 1974 to 15.2 lb per capita in 1987.

Some of the greatest changes in the U.S. diet during the past two decades have been seen in beverage use (Putnam, 1989). Between 1966 and 1987, per-capita coffee consumption decreased from 35.8 to 26.5 gal. In contrast, consumption of tea, both hot and iced, increased from 6.5 to 7.0 gal and per-capita consumption of soft drinks went from 17.9 gal in 1966 to 30.3 gal in 1987. The reported adult per-capita consumption of alcoholic beverages also grew from 32.1 to 40.1 gal between 1966 and 1987; declines in use of distilled spirits were countered by increases in the use of beer and wine.

Sales of snack foods increased by more than 8% in 1985, reaching a total of nearly $7.5 billion (Supermarket Business, 1986). Within this category, the greatest change since 1984 has been seen for fruit rolls and fruit bars, which increased nearly 23%. Potato chip sales have grown by more than 9% since 1984, totaling more than $1.8 billion— twice that of any other snack item. In 1985, candy and gum sales reached a total of nearly $9 billion; sales of diet, low-calorie, and sugarless candy and gum accounted for less than 1% of this total. High-calorie, high-fat gourmet foods are selling as well as some of the newer low-calorie, low-fat products. For example, sales of super-premium (higher in butterfat) ice cream increased by 20% in 1985 (Progressive Grocer, 1986).

The great growth in the number of fast-service food outlets has had a substantial effect on food consumption patterns (Capps, 1986). Potato products, cheese, tomatoes, and chicken have benefited from increased consumption away from home.

Economic and Demographic Influences on Change

From 1970 to 1985, poultry became a lower-priced alternative to red meat. Similarly, consumers switched to vegetable-based fats and oils, having been attracted to their lower prices compared with the more expensive animal-based fats and oils. In contrast, fish consumption increased, despite increases in fish prices during the same period. Price, however, probably became less of a factor in the 1980s. The trends of the 1970s and early 1980s may have been fixed in place as a result of increasing concerns about diet and health.

Historically, as real income rose, demand increased for some relatively expensive foods such as beef, poultry, shellfish, processed milk products, and vegetables (Smallwood and Blaylock, 1981). But large increases in real income are necessary to generate substantial increases in food consumption (Capps, 1986). At present, income is no longer a primary determinant of food consumption or of nutrient intake, except for those at poverty levels (Senauer, 1986). Rising real income is associated with greater demand for food products that are convenient to prepare and for meals served outside the home (Kinsey, 1983).

Demographic changes have also affected food consumption patterns. The percentage of single-person households increased from 10.9% in 1950 to 22.5% in 1980, and the proportion of households with more than two people decreased from 60.3 to 46.2% (U.S. Department of Commerce, 1983). Single-person and two-person households use more convenience foods per person than do larger households (Capps, 1986).

Age-related factors are also associated with food selection. For example, older people are more likely to eat breakfast, whereas younger people are more likely to eat meals away from home (Schoenborn and Cohen, 1986).

CHANGES IN CONSUMER ATTITUDES AND KNOWLEDGE

Not surprisingly, just as food choices are changing, so too are consumers' attitudes and beliefs about food. An emerging consensus that diet is a risk factor for major chronic diseases such as cardiovascular disease, cancer, and hypertension is influencing consumer behavior and the choices available in the marketplace.

One useful source of information on consumer attitudes toward nutrition and their food purchasing behaviors is a national survey conducted annually since 1974 by the Food Marketing Institute (FMI) entitled *Trends—Consumer Attitudes & the Supermarket*. For example, in the 1990 survey (FMI, 1990), 95% of respondents reported being "very concerned" or "somewhat concerned" about the "nutritional content" of the food they eat. The proportion of shoppers who reported being "very concerned" has held steady since 1987. People age 50 and older were more concerned about nutrition than were people between the ages of 18 and 39, and although they ranked nutrition as less important than taste or product safety, they considered it more important than price or ease of preparation. Of particular note is the increase in the proportion of shoppers (from 9% in 1983 to 46% in 1990) who indicated fat content as their primary concern about the nutritional composition of foods (FMI, 1990).

Changes in the ways that consumers prepare food have tended to reflect nutrition concerns to some extent. The 1989 *Trends* survey (FMI, 1989) revealed that among the 55% of consumers who reported that they cooked or prepared foods differently since 1984 to 1986, 37% of them were frying less, 24% were using less salt, and 20% were adding less fat to foods. Consumers who either had not changed their food preparation practices or had already incorporated these behaviors into their food preparation patterns before 1984 were not surveyed on this question. The percentage of surveyed consumers reporting that they cooked or prepared foods differently since 1985 grew to 61% in the 1990 *Trends* survey (FMI, 1990).

The Food and Drug Administration's (FDA's) Health and Diet Survey, conducted every 2 years since 1979, assesses changes in public beliefs and knowledge related to diet and health issues. In 1988, 71% of the respondents reported that they had changed their diet recently to prevent heart disease—up from 61% in 1986 (Levy et al., 1988). These data suggest that people who changed their diets did so in accordance with the principles of dietary recommendations. USDA per-capita food consumption data confirm these trends (Putnam, 1989). As noted earlier, there has been a shift toward consumption of food perceived as low in fat or calories or with other positive characteristics (e.g., increase in consumption of poultry, fish, grains and other cereal products, fresh fruits and vegetables, and low-fat milk and yogurt and a decrease in consumption of red meat and whole milk).

However, the improvements consumers are making in their eating habits are very selective, as indicated by a 1987 *New York Times* poll (Burros, 1988) based on telephone interviews with 1,870 adults nationwide. For example, consumers who decrease their intake of fat by eating smaller servings of a fatty food, such as a fatty cut of meat, may substitute a salad with 5 to 6 tablespoons of salad dressing, resulting in consumption of more fat and fewer nutrients. Food disappearance data support this conclusion (see Table 3-1), showing increased consumption of fats and oils (primarily from vegetable sources) between 1970 and 1987. According to a survey by *American Health* magazine (Mothner, 1987), eating and drinking patterns in the United States are changing to meet the needs of different situations, and specific foods believed to confer unique benefits are being selected.

Is the U.S. public selective, or is it confused? The FDA's Health and Diet Surveys (Levy et al., 1988) include several questions related to consumer knowledge. In 1988, for example, 35% of those surveyed considered dietary fat as a risk factor for high blood pressure as compared with only 6% in 1979. As of 1988, 25% considered dietary fat as a risk factor for cancer. From 1979 to 1982, when the National Heart, Lung, and Blood Institute (NHLBI) and FDA launched an initiative to inform the public about the relationship between sodium intake and hypertension, there was a 300% increase in respondents who mentioned sodium as a risk factor for hypertension. The Health and Diet Surveys also indicated that during the highly visible advertising campaign for Kellogg All-Bran cereal (1984 to 1986), there was a 350% increase in respondents who mentioned fiber as a factor that might help to prevent cancer.

The percentage of people who perceive dietary fats as a risk factor for heart disease rose from 29% in 1983 to 55% in 1988. The mention of cholesterol as a risk factor for heart disease increased similarly. On the other hand, these surveys indicated that respondents did not understand which kinds of foods contain cholesterol, what the term *cholesterol-free* means, whether vegetable oil contains saturated or unsaturated fat, and whether some fats are higher in calories than others. Seventy percent of respondents to the 1988 Health and Diet Survey were either not sure or believed that all foods containing fat had cholesterol. Forty percent of the respondents thought that a food containing vegetable oil or labeled cholesterol-free would also be low in saturated fat; another 20% of the respondents were not sure what cholesterol-free implied about the saturated fat content of a food. Only 20% of the population realized that all fats have essentially the same number of calories. In short, it appears that much of the public equates cholesterol with saturated fat, which is "bad," while anything free of cholesterol is equated with low saturated fat, which is "good" (Levy et al., 1988). Yet less than 20% of the respondents knew that hydrogenation made fat more saturated, and only 27% had ever heard of monounsaturated fat. Moreover, 65% of the population questioned by the FDA in 1988 did not know that polyunsaturated fats are more likely than saturated fats to be liquid.

These data suggest that the public is highly concerned about diet and health but is lacking the detailed knowledge needed to act effectively on these concerns. Another interpretation of the data is that the public, however concerned, does not wish to become knowledgeable in biochemistry in order to eat well. The challenge then becomes not to try to teach them more than they want to know but to give information that will allow them to make health-promoting food choices based on some easily comprehended rules. This information should be packaged in ways that fit into the busy lives of people. Finally, people experience the pull of many interests and motivations that compete with eating healthfully, and most people are reluctant to make drastic changes in life-style (Light et al., 1989). The relationships between such attitudes and motivations and dietary behavior are explored in greater detail in the following section.

THEORIES OF ATTITUDE AND BEHAVIOR CHANGE

The ultimate goal in implementing dietary recommendations is to produce desirable behavior changes. Such changes can result from a variety of causes—both environmental and internal. For example, a person may shift to a lower-fat diet because of a change in the food supply (an environmental cause) or because of new beliefs about the role of fat in the diet or the acquisition of new food preparation skills (internal causes). Since it is unlikely that implementation strategies can rely on environmental changes alone, it is important to examine the role of internal factors in influencing human behavior.

Two major approaches to behavior change that rely on internal factors are the communication/persuasion model and the social learning model. Some understanding of the findings of basic research on influencing human behavior may help to guard against either overly optimistic or overly pessimistic assessments of the prospects for changing eating habits to promote health.

Communication/Persuasion Model

The communication/persuasion model focuses on modifying attitudes as a means of changing behavior. Attitudes are people's general predispositions to evaluate other people, objects, and issues either favorably or unfavorably. The attitudes relevant to implementing dietary recommendations range from general attitudes about changing diets for health purposes (i.e., is it perceived to be a worthwhile idea or not?) to attitudes toward specific foods (e.g., do I like premium ice cream?). This construct has achieved a preeminent position because of the assumption that attitude change is an important mediating variable between the acquisition of new knowledge and behavioral change (see reviews by Chaiken and Stangor, 1987; Cialdini et al., 1981; and Cooper and Croyle, 1984). That is, new knowledge (e.g., saturated fat raises cholesterol levels) is believed to produce new attitudes (e.g., saturated fat is bad), which in turn produces new behavior (e.g., avoidance of foods high in saturated fat).

Attitude Change Theories

Early theories of persuasion were based on the assumption that effective influence required a sequence of steps (see, for example, McGuire, 1985 and Strong, 1925). A first step typically was *exposure* of a person to some new information, from a single channel of communication or through multiple channels such as face-to-face confrontations, the mass media, programs at work sites and churches, and in-store food displays. Second, people must *attend* to the information presented. Because literally hundreds of messages compete for people's attention each day, relatively few are successful in attracting it (Bogart, 1967). A third step is *reception*, which involves the storage of selected information segments in long-term memory. Just because a person is consciously aware of an informational presentation, there is no guarantee that any aspect of what has been seen and heard will create more than a fleeting impression.

Likewise, just because some new information is learned as a result of an educational campaign, there is no guarantee that this knowledge will lead to attitude or behavior change. Current research strongly indicates that attitude change depends upon the manner in which the information is interpreted, evaluated, and *elaborated* so that it makes some sense to the person. The more favorable the cognitive or affective response to the information, the more likely that attitudes will change in a positive direction. Once the information received has elicited various thoughts or feelings, these responses must be *integrated* into an overall evaluation or attitude capable of guiding subsequent *action* (Petty and Cacioppo, 1984).

A change early in this proposed sequence will not inevitably lead to a change later on, because each step in the sequence may be viewed as a conditional probability. Thus, even if the likelihood of achieving each step is 60%, the probability of achieving all six steps (exposure, attention, reception, elaboration, integration, and action) would be $.60^6$ or only 5% (McGuire, 1989).

Another reason why a change early in the sequence may not lead to a change in a later stage is because some steps in the sequence may be independent of each other. For example, although a person's ability to learn and recall new information (e.g., facts about nutrition or diet and health) was often believed to be an important causal determinant of, and prerequisite to, attitude and behavior change, little empirical evidence has accumulated to support this view (McGuire, 1985; Petty and Cacioppo, 1981). Rather, evidence shows that message learning can occur in the absence of attitude change and that people's attitudes may change in the absence of learning the specific information presented. For example, consider two people who hear that the consumption of oat bran can reduce one's cholesterol level and reduce the risk of heart disease. One person, who is overweight and constantly dieting, responds to this information with the thought that oat bran must be good for one's health. Later that week in the supermarket, the person passes the cereal aisle and selects an oat bran product because it is perceived as a diet food that will help the person to lose weight. In this instance, the original information about the link between the product and heart disease was lost, but the self-generated (and probably mistaken) elaborations or translation of that information (from disease prevention to healthful to diet) guides the behavior. Another person hears the same information and responds with the thought that there is no need to be concerned since there is no family history of heart disease. Next week in the supermarket, this person passes over the oat bran products, even though there is a perfect recall of the original information that was presented. Since the person does not feel personally vulnerable, learning the new information has no effect on that person's behavior.

Current psychological theories of influence focus on how and why various features of the persuasive communication (e.g., the message source, its content, and method of presentation) affect each of the steps in the communication sequence. The most work by far, however, addresses the ways that variables affect the elaboration stage of information processing. This stage is sometimes viewed as the most critical, since it is during this stage that the presented information achieves meaning, is evaluated favorably or unfavorably, and is accepted or rejected.

Models of the processes that occur during the elaboration stage emphasize one of two relatively distinct routes to persuasion (Chaiken, 1987; Petty and Cacioppo, 1981, 1986; Sherman, 1987). The first, or central route, involves cognitive activity whereby the person draws upon experience and knowledge to scrutinize and evaluate carefully the issue-relevant information presented in the communication. For this to occur, the person must possess sufficient motivation, ability, and opportunity to think about the perceived merits of the information provided. The end result of this processing is an attitude that is well articulated and integrated into the person's belief structure. Attitudes changed in this way are relatively persistent, predictive of behavior, and resistant to change until they are challenged by cogent contrary information (Petty and Cacioppo, 1986). Using a biological analogy, McGuire (1964) suggests that just as people can be made more resistant to disease by giving them a mild form of a germ, people can be made more resistant to attacks on their attitudes by inoculating their new opinions. The inoculation treatment consists of exposing people to a few pieces of attacking information and showing them how to refute it. People whose attitudes are bolstered with inoculation treatments become less vulnerable to subsequent attacks on their attitudes than do people whose attitudes are bolstered with supportive information alone (McGuire and Papageorgis, 1961).

Attitudes may also be changed by a *peripheral route* in which simple cues in the persuasion context either elicit an affective state (e.g., happiness) that becomes associated with the advocated position (as in classical conditioning) (Staats and Staats, 1958) or trigger a relatively simple inference or rule that the person can use to judge the validity of the message (Chaiken, 1987). Advertisers attempt to use this strategy when they associate a food product with good times and fun or when they invoke a simple inference such as, "A doctor said it, so it must be true." Changes induced by this peripheral route have been found to be less persistent and predictive of behavior than changes based on more extensive thought about the merits of the arguments in the message. Thus, a person who develops a negative attitude toward salt simply because his or her doctor said it was bad is likely to be less in compliance with the appropriate dietary regimen over the long term than is a person who developed a negative attitude toward salt after careful reflection upon the personal consequences of, and reasons for, the doctor's recommendation.

Links Between Attitudes and Behaviors

Once a person's attitude has changed, it is important that one's new attitude rather than the old habits guide behavior. A considerable amount of research has addressed the links between attitudes and behavior, and many situational and dispositional factors have been shown to enhance the consistency between them. Attitudes have been found to have a greater impact on behavior when, for example, (1) people are of a certain personality type (e.g., those who tend not to follow the opinions of others), (2) the attitudes are consistent with the person's underlying beliefs, (3) the attitudes are based on extensive amounts of issue-relevant knowledge or personal experience, (4) the attitudes were formed as a result of issue-relevant thinking, and (5) cues indicate that the person's attitude is relevant to the behavior (see Ajzen, 1989 for a comprehensive review).

Two general types of theories regarding the process by which attitudes guide health-related behavior have achieved widespread acceptance. One of them focuses on thoughtful reasoning processes, whereas the other type focuses on more automatic processes. A good example of the first type of theory is Ajzen and Fishbein's (1980) *theory of reasoned action*, which assumes that "people consider the implications of their actions before they decide to engage or not engage in a given behavior" (p. 5). According to this theory, people form intentions to perform or not to perform behaviors, and these intentions are based on the person's attitude toward the behaviors as well as perceptions of the opinions of others (norms). This theory focuses on the perceived likelihood that certain benefits will accrue or costs will be avoided and on the desirability (or aversiveness) of those benefits (or costs).

The specific beliefs that are relevant to taking recommended health actions have been outlined in the *health belief model* (Rosenstock, 1974). These include beliefs about (1) one's personal susceptibility to some disorder, (2) the perceived severity of the disorder, (3) the subjective benefits of engaging in a recommended action, and (4) the costs (e.g., financial and psychological) of engaging in the behavior. That is, people are assumed to engage in health-related actions to the extent that they believe that some health concern is relevant to them and that the likely effectiveness and other benefits of the recommended action outweigh its costs. The reasoned-action theories have proven remarkably successful in accounting for a wide variety of behaviors (Janz and Becker, 1984; Sheppard et al., 1988).

In contrast to these theories of reasoned action, Fazio (1990) has proposed an *accessibility theory*, which suggests that much behavior is spontaneous and that attitudes guide behavior by a relatively automatic process. Specifically, Fazio argues that attitudes can guide behavior without any deliberate reflection or reasoning if the attitude (1) is highly accessible (i.e., comes to mind spontaneously by the mere presence of the attitude object) and (2) influences the perception of the object—i.e., if the attitude is favorable (or unfavorable), the qualities of the object appear favorable (or unfavorable). For example, when confronted with a dish of ice cream, positive feelings may come to mind automatically, thus causing the ice cream to appear more desirable and leading the person to consume the food. The various costs and benefits of eating the ice cream may not be considered at all or may be weighed only after the food is eaten.

The theory proposed by Fazio suggests some conditions under which the reasoned or the more spontaneous attitude processes occur. He notes that factors related to motivation, ability, and opportunity will be important in determining the means by which attitudes guide behavior. Thus, for behavioral decisions that are perceived to have serious personal consequences, attitudes are likely to guide behavior by a deliberate process of reflection, but when consequences are perceived to be less serious, spontaneous attitude activation should be more important. Similarly, as the time allowed for decision making is reduced, the importance of spontaneous attitude activation processes should be increased over more deliberative processes. A typical shopper in a supermarket is confronted with many choices for every category of food and has a limited time to reach a decision. This environment is not likely to foster much cogitation. Rather, simple cues (e.g., packaging), old habits, and well-ingrained attitudes (rather than relatively new and less accessible ones) are likely to guide choices. Much can be done, however, to simplify the decision-making environment (e.g., simple shelf labeling) and to provoke thought before selection (e.g., in-store health displays) so that one's new attitudes rather than one's old habits are more likely to guide behavior.

Social Learning Model

Models of attitude change focus on persuading people to adopt new beliefs and evaluations in order to change behavior. In some areas, the implications of a new attitude for behavior are relatively straightforward and simple to implement (e.g., preference and voting for a particular candidate in an upcoming election). Changes in attitude related to diet and health are an important first step but may be insufficient to produce the desired behavioral responses. People may also need to acquire new skills and self-perceptions that allow newly acquired attitudes and intentions to be translated into action. Furthermore, once an attitude has yielded a new behavior, this new behavior may not persist in the absence of incentives.

Bandura's (1977, 1986) *social* (cognitive) *learning theory* provides a framework for understanding these processes. This theory is based on evidence of a reciprocal linkage of a person's cognitions with both the person's behavior and the environment. Importantly, from the perspective of the social learning theory, the power of vicariously experienced and self-generated consequences in controlling action is recognized. As in the theory of reasoned action and the health belief model, described above, voluntary behavior in the social learning model is determined by the anticipated consequences of various courses of action (Rosenstock et al., 1988). These anticipations of rewards or punishments may be based on personal experience, on the observed experiences of others, or on cognitive reasoning processes. An individual's beliefs about the consequences of behavior can be more influential than the actual consequences in determining what actions are selected, and people are viewed as being capable of providing their own rewards and punishments for their actions (self-regulation).

Importantly, before behavior can be changed, it may first be necessary for the person to learn new actions (skills) or new sequences of already acquired actions. For example, a person may have developed a negative attitude toward saturated fat but does not have the food preparation skills required to eat less of it. New skills may be acquired through direct experience or through observations of the behavior patterns of others (modeling). The most effective models are people who are admired or people with whom individuals identify. However, people do not always behave in ways consonant with known behaviors. That is, learning (or knowledge) does not guarantee that the person will engage in the behavior that has been learned, because various incentives (both external and intrinsic) may be necessary to translate knowledge into action.

One particularly important cognitive determinant of whether knowledge and attitudes have behavioral implications concerns people's assessments of their own capabilities (their judgments of *self-efficacy*) (Bandura, 1982). People assess their capabilities in a variety of ways, e.g., by assessing their own accomplishments and performances or their current physiological state, by observing and comparing their behaviors with those of other people, and by considering the expectations and norms set for themselves by other people in their lives. Judgments of self-efficacy are important because extensive research indicates that the higher the level of perceived efficacy, the more likely people are to persist in a new, learned behavior (e.g., preparing and eating low-fat foods). Of the various ways to influence self-efficacy, provision of guided practice and specific skills training (e.g., teaching people how to improve their supermarket shopping skills or practicing specific cooking methods) has proven to be especially powerful (Meyer and Henderson, 1974). Thus, an important procedure for instilling self-efficacy is to set relatively small and easily accomplished goals initially (e.g., change one's breakfast menu for the next week), and as self-efficacy increases, provide more challenging goals (e.g., change one's dinner habits). This procedure is based on the theory that the satisfaction derived from subgoal attainment can build intrinsic interest in the task at hand, thereby leading to persisting change.

Implications of Theoretical Perspectives for Changing Diet for Health

Although evidence has shown that it is possible to improve people's knowledge of food and nutrition, this new knowledge does not invariably result in attitude and behavior changes (Axelson et al., 1985). Information will be successful in producing relatively enduring changes in attitudes and behavior only if people are motivated and able to process the information and if this processing results in favorable cognitive and affective reactions. Furthermore, once attitudes have changed, implementation of change may require learning new behavioral skills and developing feelings of self-efficacy.

Although some attitudes are based on a careful reasoning process, others are formed as a result of relatively simple cues in the persuasive message or the surrounding context. There are important consequences of the manner of attitude change, such as whether or not the attitude change will last. For example, it is possible to change attitudes without providing an extensive informational campaign, but the resulting attitudes are likely to be less stable and directive of behavior. Finally, just as some attitudes are thoughtfully based whereas others are not, some behaviors are the product of deliberate reflection on costs and benefits, but others are much more spontaneous.

Since implementation of dietary recommendations necessitates long-lasting changes in attitudes with behavioral consequences, the central route to persuasion appears to be the preferred influence strategy. Unfortunately, this is not simple. The recipient of the new information must have the motivation, ability, and opportunity to process the new information. One of the most important determinants of motivation to think about a message is the perceived personal relevance of that message. When personal relevance is great, people are motivated to scrutinize the information presented and to integrate it with their beliefs, but when there is little perceived relevance, messages may be ignored or processed for peripheral cues, such as whether or not the source of the communication is attractive. Perceived personal vulnerability to some threat has been found to be a particularly important determinant of preventive health beliefs and behaviors (Janz and Becker, 1984). Yet many young people in the U.S. population, for example, may believe that health messages about food are not aimed at them or have few consequences for them. An important goal of any implementation strategy should be to increase people's motivation to process messages about diet and health by increasing the perceived personal relevance of these messages. That is, the issue of diet and health must become relevant to more people than just those in high-risk populations.

Even people motivated to think about diet and health messages must respond to these messages with favorable cognitive and affective reactions before there can be long-lasting changes in attitudes with behavioral consequences. Different types of information will elicit different responses in various segments of the population. Since attitudes toward food are based on a variety of factors (e.g., social norms and perceived healthfulness), different types of appeals and strategies will need to be developed for the diverse targets of influence.

Messages concerning diet and health are likely to be relatively complex and therefore difficult to assimilate and implement. Unlike some preventive health messages focused on only one attitude that is to be changed (e.g., cigarettes are bad, so don't smoke), messages on diet and health require considerable sophistication to process. Multiple attitudes are involved, and it is generally inappropriate to label certain foods as invariably bad. Much research is needed to determine the level of complexity at which messages can be presented to different audiences and the type of information that would elicit positive reactions.

Even if the relevant attitudes are changed, the new attitudes cannot influence behavior if they do not come to mind before the opportunity for action is presented or if people lack the necessary skills or confidence to implement them. People will need to be encouraged to think before they eat so that the new attitudes will come to mind. They must also acquire the behavioral skills needed to implement their new attitudes.

People may form positive attitudes toward low-fat entrees as the result of an educational campaign, but if the first low-fat meal they try in their workplace cafeteria is unpleasant, two different evaluations are formed—"low-fat food is good for you" and "low-fat food tastes bad." Since beliefs and attitudes based on direct experiences come to mind more readily than do attitudes that are based solely on externally provided information, the effectiveness of the information favorable to low-fat food (even if it comes to mind eventually) is severely attenuated (Fazio and Zanna, 1981). Consistent with social learning theory, various procedures for enhancing self-efficacy such as skills training, self-regulation, and reinforcement may be needed in order to maintain behaviors that reflect a person's new attitudes.

COMMUNICATION THROUGH THE MEDIA

The two models described in the previous section—the communication/persuasion model and the social learning model—rely heavily on the media to influence behavior. It is therefore appropriate at this point to describe briefly the components and functions of the media. The following section provides examples of the media being used in schools, work sites, and communities to improve dietary patterns. Several of the committee's recommended strategies and actions to implement dietary recommendations, described in Chapters 5 through 8, involve the use of the media.

The media are used frequently to inform, educate, and motivate health-seeking individuals and members of communities to improve their dietary behaviors. This may occur in relatively informal ways (e.g., health promotion messages in magazines or television shows) or in planned campaigns as described in the next section. The media are a principal source of information on food and nutrition for many people. Because the success of the media in influencing consumer knowledge and behavior is widely acknowledged, it will continue to play an important role in any comprehensive efforts to improve the diets and health of the U.S. population. The committee uses the term media to refer to broadcast media such as radio and television; print media such as newspapers, magazines, and brochures; and newer forms of communication such as videos and computer programs.

Two major functions of the mass media are to inform and persuade. Recent incidents have demonstrated clear links between coverage of an issue and consumer response. Extensive media coverage of a report claiming that children were being excessively exposed to pesticides and other agricultural chemicals, particularly from Alar on apples, led to a large drop in apple consumption (Smith, 1990) and helped to reduce consumer confidence in the safety of the food supply (FMI, 1989, 1990). In another example, increased sales of Kellogg high-fiber All-Bran cereal resulted from advertising the product with the National Cancer Institute's message that high-fiber diets may reduce the risk of colon cancer (Freimuth et al., 1988; Levy and Stokes, 1987). The FDA, reporting the results of its 1979 to 1988 Health and Diet Surveys, noted that increased public knowledge of diet and disease relationships "seems to occur during periods when the diet/disease messages gain access to the mass media" (Levy et al., 1988). It added that the increased media coverage that effected these gains in public awareness was primarily due to "intensified and coordinated health promotion efforts by industry, government and the scientific community."

The four broad sectors of society addressed in this report—public, private, health-care professions, and education (Chapters 5 to 8)—use the media as a tool to communicate their messages on diet and health because of the media's ability to reach many people in a cost-effective manner. Media access is often purchased, but it may be available at no charge if the media decide that a particular activity or initiative is newsworthy or that it should be promoted as a public service. To interest the media in promoting dietary recommendations, implementors must find ways to make the messages continually appealing and newsworthy, since the media present material that they believe will attract and interest consumers and thereby enhance their ability to attract funds and advertisers. Therefore, implementors should learn, for example, to write effective press releases, provide accurate and useful background material, and offer spokespersons for interviews.

The media can also provide instruction and illustrations on how to make and maintain desirable behavior changes. This function of the media needs to be marshaled by implementors in communities across the United States. Media attention to dietary recommendations and their implementation is likely to be most effective in improving eating behaviors when the messages can be integrated and coordinated with other community health promotion efforts such as face-to-face instruction in classes, incentive programs at work sites, and widespread availability of health-promoting foods at restaurants. One particularly challenging task for implementors will be to use the media in more innovative ways to improve the health-related behaviors of the difficult-to-reach segments of the population, including low-income, poorly educated, low-literacy, and some minority groups. To reach these groups, implementors will need to adapt their messages to make them culturally specific and personally relevant (Freimuth, 1990; Freimuth and Mettger, 1990; Nickens, 1990; White and Maloney, 1990). Difficult-to-reach people are most likely to understand and accept messages that are simple, concrete, and "adapted sensitively to the target audience's cultural beliefs" (Freimuth, 1990, p. 181). The messages should probably emphasize immediate rather than long-term benefits from adopting healthy behaviors and be constructed so as to stimulate interest in the subject. Dissemination of information through printed brochures and pamphlets is not likely to be very effective with groups that tend to be infrequent readers and have poor reading skills.

REVIEW OF EVIDENCE ON CHANGING DIET TO BENEFIT HEALTH

Because of the many complexities involved, public policy initiated to modify diet to benefit health should call for the use of the communication/persuasion and social learning models. Information regarding diet and health (communication inputs) can and should come from a variety of sources, including the mass media, face-to-face interactions, community events (e.g., health fairs and contests to provide incentives to change), and from alterations in the environment (e.g., provision and clear display of health-promoting food choices in schools and retail food establishments).

As shown in Table 3-2, communication roles differ for the sender (the educator) and the recipient (the learner). The sender begins by determining the receiver's needs so that the appropriate information can be presented. The sender must next set a new agenda by gaining the attention of the receiver, a step analogous to the town crier's "Now hear ye." In modern times, the social marketing approach can awaken interest by a variety of means and messages that create a sense that the issue (e.g., nutrition) is personally relevant. The sender's next two steps provide the factual information needed, coupled with incentives for the receiver to make changes.

The first three steps shown for the receiver are the essence of the communication/persuasion model. The receiver first becomes aware of the information and may end up with changed beliefs and atti-

TABLE 3-2 The Communication/Persuasion–Social Learning Formulation

Communication Functions for the Sender (listed in desired sequence)
Determine receiver's needs
Set agenda (gain attention)
Provide information
Provide incentives
Provide training
Provide cues to action, including environmental change
Provide support and self-management skills

Target Objectives for the Receiver (listed in desired sequence)
Exposure to and awareness of communication
Reception of message and knowledge change
Change in interest, thinking, motives, and attitudes
Learn and practice new skills
Take action and assess outcomes
Maintain action, practice self-management skills
Become an opinion leader
Give feedback to sender

tudes if the persuasion is successful. These changed attitudes and beliefs render the person more open to behavior modification attempts. The next three steps are the essence of the social learning model. Once attitudes are changed, people are motivated to learn new skills to achieve and maintain behavior change. In the last two steps, the receiver becomes a transmitter and advocate.

Although there is an extensive literature on efforts to produce dietary change for the purpose of weight reduction, there are fewer studies of educational interventions designed to produce qualitative dietary change, i.e., changes in the types of foods consumed; and only some of these describe precisely the type and amount of education provided. This section reviews more than 50 studies reported in the past two decades that have evaluated the effectiveness of nutrition education in producing qualitative dietary changes in either special subgroups or the general population. The results of these studies provide insights into what succeeds (and what fails) and suggest the amount, type, and duration of education needed to achieve important beneficial changes in eating habits.

The following types of studies are reviewed: small-group classroom studies; programs that activate social support systems; school-based programs for adolescents; health communication at points of purchase; studies conducted at work sites; regional and national mass media campaigns; and comprehensive, integrated community-based multifactor risk-reduction programs. The first six types of studies are potential components of community-based interventions, which are reviewed later in the chapter.

Small-Group Classroom Studies

In small-group classroom studies, face-to-face communication has generally been combined with supplementary printed materials to teach selected groups of adults, often those at high risk for developing health problems because of their life-styles or the presence of other risk factors of interest to the investigators (Meyer and Henderson, 1974; MRFIT Research Group, 1982). These studies have shown that education based on social learning and self-directed change is more effective than the more traditional method of imparting knowledge alone (Bandura, 1986; Meyer and Henderson, 1974). Programs that provide not only the information needed to change knowledge and attitudes but also instruction in methods of monitoring change and guidance on how to achieve *gradual* incremental change in dietary habits have been successful, for example, in lowering blood cholesterol levels (Arntzenius et al., 1985; Bruno et al., 1983; Carmody et al., 1986; Glanz, 1985; Hjermann et al., 1981; Meyer and Henderson, 1974; MRFIT Research Group, 1982; Puska, 1985; Wilhelmsen et al., 1986). Educational programs relying largely on self-help printed instructions that include the social learning features mentioned above have also been successful in lowering cholesterol levels by dietary means for adult participants identified as being at high risk for cardiovascular disease (Crouch et al., 1986). An increasing number of small-group studies in such high-risk adults have been conducted in different cultural groups in various countries and have reported effecting lasting changes in dietary habits.

A limitation of these studies is that their subjects were motivated to participate in them through screening tests that identified such factors as high blood cholesterol levels that placed subjects at high risk for cardiovascular disease. Some effective methods of reaching the general public, including those who will not volunteer for repeated classroom sessions, have been developed and are reported later in this chapter.

Programs That Activate Social Support Systems

Direct or indirect social support can help bring about dietary change, especially when information and role models are provided to the many people who are not strongly motivated to seek either personal counseling or group classroom instruction.

Such support can be provided, for example, by television, which is an increasing force in the dissemination of new commercial, political, or religious ideas to individuals linked to the media source but not usually to each other. Nevertheless, traditional networks of peers and family members that provide two-way communication are still the strongest influence on the individual, especially when the safety and good sense of a recommended novel approach to life-style and health are questioned, as reviewed by Rogers (1983). These traditional networks can be regarded as guardians of existing social norms that can clearly act as barriers to behavior change; however, they can also be activated to promote the adoption of new and beneficial health practices and are, thus, a potentially important resource.

Through health communication programs, potential leaders from the general population can be identified to serve as informal health educators within their peer networks. In the Finnish North Karelia Project, for example, such individuals were recruited and, after a brief 4-hour training session, became a useful part of the program. Using face-to-face channels, they helped to communicate the project's goals, including a wide array of desirable dietary changes (Puska et al., 1986).

Groups recruited from the general population on the basis of shared attributes, such as having a high risk of a particular disease, may also become effective communicators of health messages. In the Stanford Three-Community Study, for example, health educators gave a group of high-risk adults approximately 20 hours of intensive instruction in self-directed change (see more detailed discussion of this study later in this chapter). In comparison with other members of the adult population, those subjects were found to converse with a larger number of their acquaintances more frequently on health topics (Meyer et al., 1977). Those at equivalent high risk who were not exposed to this special education were not activated to spread the message. Subjects in this study exposed to a mass media health education campaign were more likely to become opinion leaders (or unofficial health educators, so to speak) if they felt personally involved by virtue of completing a lengthy survey in which they identified their personal cardiovascular disease-risk status (Meyer et al., 1977).

Given this evidence for the spontaneous creation of opinion leaders as a function of the degree of exposure to health education and of perceived personal relevance, one can see why a popularly conceived and implemented health communication program applied to any part of a system (such as a school, a work site, or a community) can lead to at least some dissemination of information and potential for behavior change in individuals within that system. Any individual exposed to such an education program is therefore a potential participant in the spread of a health message.

Results from family-centered programs buttress the view that social support enhances individual instruction and elicits dietary change (Arntzenius et al., 1985; Bruno et al., 1983; Carmody et al., 1982; Ehnholm et al., 1982; Glanz, 1985; Hjermann et al., 1981; Meyer and Henderson, 1974; Nader et al., 1986; Perry et al., 1989; Puska, 1985; Wilhelmsen et al., 1986).

Social support networks are varied and numerous. To provide optimal health communication, one must first use the most effective natural networks (Rogers, 1983). For example, birth control practices and agricultural innovations diffuse through different networks in the same community (Marshall, 1971). Nutrition education will have its own natural network that can be identified through social marketing methods, such as the use of focus groups that bring 10 to 20 individuals together to learn who they talk to and rely on for sources of opinion in matters of diet and health (Kotler and Zaltmann, 1971).

School-Based Programs for Adolescents

Through school-based programs, information can be channeled to peer networks of young children and adolescents. They have therefore been used in numerous health communication studies, most notably in highly successful attempts to prevent smoking among adolescents (Best et al., 1988; Killen, 1985; Telch et al., 1982). School-based programs administered to groups of tenth graders in two different areas of northern California have also resulted in self-reported decreases in saturated fat and cholesterol intake from snack foods (King et al., 1988) and statements from students that they would choose more "heart-healthy" snacks (Killen et al., 1988). The approximately 7 hours of diet and nutrition instruction in this broadly focused health course was divided almost equally among general nutrition information, skills training for change, and skills training to prevent a return to previous habits. Special attention was paid to making the information personally relevant (fostering the central route of attitude change) and to providing guided practice in menu planning, identifying high-risk foods, countering nutrition myths, and resisting peer pressures (following the guidelines of social learning theory).

In this same successful diet change study, training in resisting peer pressure included countering erroneous beliefs about food, providing means of identifying external sources of pressure (e.g., advertisements and friends) to make nutritionally poor choices, and guiding the students in the practice of counterarguments. Methods common to successful smoking prevention and diet change programs incorporate elements of attitude change research (e.g., enhancing personal relevance and use of McGuire's inoculation methods) and elements of Bandura's social learning theory (e.g., increasing self-confidence and mastery of skills through stepwise guided practice in new behaviors) (Bandura, 1986; McGuire and Papageorgis, 1961). These methods were also used to produce changes in dietary habits in the small-group classes for adults. Therefore, this consistency in results among both young and older people suggests that such methods are generally effective.

Reviewing 15 federally funded school-based cardiovascular risk-reduction programs, Stone (1985) concluded that the next urgent step is to provide guidance to the investigators on how to *disseminate* school curricula focusing on dietary change. Methods should be developed (1) to recruit or persuade the school system of the wisdom of *adopting* tested curricula, (2) to train the teachers in *teaching* from these curricula, and (3) to *maintain* the quality of the curricula (Best, 1989; Stone et al., 1989). Kreuter et al. (1984) had earlier advocated a similar plan. Effective school-based curricula are available, but the many barriers to their widespread adoption must be overcome by extensive planning, training, and monitoring.

Health Communication at Points of Purchase

Modification of environmental cues in schools, work sites, restaurants, and grocery stores in a manner consistent with the social learning theory of Bandura (1977) has produced some observable but transitory changes toward health-promoting food choices (Glanz and Mullis, 1988). Tactics include provision of more such choices accompanied by easily visible labeling, altered shelf displays, and nutrition information through posters and brochures.

The most extensive point-of-purchase study in health education was conducted by investigators in the Minnesota Heart Health Program (Mullis et al., 1987). The meat industry cooperated in this effort by increasing supplies of lean meats and by training meat department personnel to aid consumers in identifying lean meat products (Mullis and Pirie, 1988). Overall, modest gains in knowledge and slight changes in behavior were observed as a result of the program, but both knowledge and behavior changes were often transitory. Because of the short-term effect of this program, Glanz and Mullis (1988) concluded that point-of-purchase education should be part of a larger campaign to be most effective.

Recently, Ellison et al. (1989) reported a 20% decline in saturated fat intake among students in boarding high schools following a training program for food service workers to modify the food served in the schools' dining halls. The main purpose of this point-of-consumption study was to show that such an environmental change can produce dietary change in the absence of a student educational component. Despite this lack, student satisfaction with the food provided was unchanged.

Studies Conducted at Work Sites

Work sites offer excellent opportunities for nutrition education. They provide a convenient locale for small-group classes for adults and allow for activation of a support system through the social networks of the work site. As in schools, there are also opportunities for changing cafeteria policies (e.g., providing point-of-purchase education) and for fostering changes to build a healthy work force.

Sallis et al. (1986) reported that approximately 50 work-site programs have been evaluated in the United States in the past decade. Many of these seem to have been effective in achieving at least short-term improvements in various life-styles and risk factor profiles, especially among high-risk individuals in programs designed to foster change in more than one risk factor, including diet.

Unfortunately, many work-site interventions are incompletely described. Successful programs have usually incorporated the self-directed change aspects of social learning theory to bring about dietary change, weight control, or smoking cessation (Blair et al., 1986; Bruno et al., 1983; Glanz, 1985; Klesges et al., 1986; Meyer and Henderson, 1974; Sallis et al., 1986; Stunkard et al., 1985; Wilbur, 1983). Reviewing such work-site programs, Glanz (1985) concluded that those which were most effective also contained changes in regulations (such as smoking policies) and the work environment (such as the inclusion of lower-fat menus in company cafeterias) (see also Glanz and Seewald-Klein, 1986). Fostering of competition among employees has increased the success of programs designed to achieve smoking cessation (Klesges et al., 1986), but there are no reports of contests used in dietary change programs.

An important challenge is whether the sequenced pattern of instruction on self-directed change can be incorporated into nutrition education programs that rely largely on use of the media, thereby decreasing costs. One study has shown considerable reductions in blood cholesterol levels and in self-reported saturated fat intake among adults in widely dispersed work sites (Miller et al., 1988). This study provided a single videotaped instruction session to groups of employees at many widely separated locations. These individuals were linked by telephone to a central computer, which provided guidance in stepwise changes to improve eating behaviors. Printed instructions were mailed to each participant following each telephone contact. These instructions were made personally relevant by linking the results of a self-administered test of dietary practices with the risk of heart attack and stroke.

Regional and National Mass Media Campaigns

Many investigators have concluded that mass media campaigns (generally based on brief radio and television announcements or spots), although useful for increasing knowledge and changing attitudes, are not usually effective in producing large and lasting behavior change unless they are linked to more comprehensive campaigns (Atkin, 1979; Farquhar et al., 1977, 1985a; Glanz, 1985; Hewitt and Blaine, 1984; McGuire, 1964; Meyer et al., 1977; Puska, 1985; Puska et al., 1981; Roberts and Maccoby, 1985; Rootman, 1985; WHO, 1986). If they are comprehensive and well conceived, however, mass media efforts may have considerable impact.

The 3-year Stanford Three-Community Study was the first community-based cardiovascular disease prevention program conducted in the United States (Farquhar et al., 1977). The communities were three semirural towns in northern California (economies centered largely around agriculture and related business) with populations of approximately 15,000 each, in which random samples of 500 people from each town were surveyed to determine their knowledge of cardiovascular disease and risk factor levels (smoking rates, body weight, blood cholesterol, and blood pressure). One community, the control, received only the yearly surveys. The two others were exposed to a mass media campaign involving frequent television and radio spots (five times a day, one of approximately 60 different public service announcements were delivered on radio and television), two weekly newspaper columns, and large quantities of mailed booklets containing heart-healthy recipes and specific information on nutrition, exercise, and weight control. The study included several unique features: (1) Educational materials were disseminated through multiple communication channels (e.g., radio, television, newspapers, mass mailings of brief notices and of detailed self-help manuals, billboards, and bus posters); (2) all educational materials were based on the attitude change and social learning elements described earlier; and (3) special means of achieving personal relevance were included (e.g., an hour-long television heart health test provided viewers with an assessment of risks derived from their personal habits of diet, exercise, and smoking, and yearly surveys provided a subset of the population with extra information on their risk factors—blood pressure and blood cholesterol levels). One of the two treatment communities was provided with a 3-month-long series of 10 lessons given to small classes of high-risk adults (Meyer and Henderson, 1974; Meyer et al., 1977). The study was evaluated through repeated yearly surveys of the 1,500 people surveyed at the baseline. In the two cities exposed to the mass media campaign, there were approximately 30% decreases in self-reported saturated fat and cholesterol intake and also significant but modest decreases of about 3% in blood cholesterol levels. Greater changes in dietary patterns and blood cholesterol levels were observed in those who received classroom instruction in addition to the mass media exposure (Farquhar et al., 1977; Fortmann et al., 1981; Maccoby et al., 1977). These findings reinforce the conclusion that behavior change is more likely in people given evidence of personal relevance.

Comprehensive, Integrated Community-Based Multifactor Risk-Reduction Programs

Several community-based health communication studies that include dietary change as a goal have been reported or are under way. The two best-known projects are the Stanford Three-Community Study discussed in the preceding section and the Finnish North Karelia Project (Puska, 1985; Puska et al., 1979, 1981, 1986; Tuomilehto et al., 1986), which both began in 1972.

The Finnish study was conducted in two adjoining counties, one of which received education through multiple communication channels in ways similar to that of the Stanford Three-Community Study. The changes in cholesterol, blood pressure, and smoking achieved after 2 and 3 years of education in the Stanford study were comparable to those achieved after the first 5 years of education in the North Karelia Project. The investigators predicted that an approximately 20 to 25% reduction in coronary events would occur in the future if the risk factor changes persisted for more than 5 years. The risk factor decreases that were achieved in the Stanford and Finnish studies for blood cholesterol, blood pressure, and smoking rates were approximately 3, 5, and 10%, respectively. In a 10-year follow-up of the Finnish study, mortality from ischemic heart disease was reduced in North Karelia (annual decrease of 2.9% among males and 4.9% among females) to a significantly greater extent compared with that in the remainder of Finland (1.9 and 3.0% annual decreases, respectively) (Tuomilehto et al., 1986).

A few other community-based studies have been conducted with educational approaches less intensive than, but similar to, those in the Stanford study and the North Karelia project. Significant changes in blood cholesterol levels, blood pressure, and smoking were found in only one of these studies, which was conducted in three small South African towns (Rossouw et al., 1981). In two others, a four-town study in Switzerland (Gutzwiller et al., 1985) and a three-town study in Australia (Egger et al., 1983), no changes in blood cholesterol levels were observed, but 6 and 9% decreases in smoking rates, respectively, were reported. The reasons for the smaller sizes of these decreases compared with those of the Stanford and Finnish studies are unclear, but it appears that the campaigns were not as extensive nor were the campaigns based on the communication/persuasion and social learning models.

Interim results of another large (total population, 350,000) and complex long-term study, the Stanford Five-City Project (Farquhar et al., 1985b, 1990), show favorable changes in smoking, blood pressure, diet, exercise, and blood cholesterol levels comparable to those achieved in the Stanford Three-Community Study (Farquhar et al., 1990). The consistency of findings of these two studies in the United States suggests that cost-effective communitywide programs (macrointerventions) are effective in achieving dietary changes in the general population, just as confidence exists that small-group classes can bring about change in certain population subgroups (microinterventions). Two additional extensive and well-evaluated studies are now in progress in the United States: the Minnesota Heart Health Program, involving six communities with a total population of 356,000 (Blackburn et al., 1984), and the Pawtucket Heart Health Study in Rhode Island, involving two cities with a total population of 173,000 (Lasater et al., 1984).

Effective Educational Methods

The effectiveness of community-based studies in decreasing the risks and incidence of cardiovascular disease is enhanced by ensuring the implementation of comprehensive programs that involve the mass media, schools, work sites, and local health organizations (Farquhar, 1985a; Lefebvre and Flora, 1988). Procedures include analysis of community resources and community needs (including needs of various subgroups within the population) as well as pretesting of various educational methods. The term *social marketing* has been applied to these methods by Kotler and Zaltman (1971), Manoff (1985), and Lefebvre and Flora (1988).

It is helpful to conduct formal tests of effectiveness in small groups before applying methods in large field studies. For example, the Stanford Three-Community Study investigators developed some intensive instruction methods that followed Bandura's methods of self-directed change (Bandura, 1977) and applied them to 36 high-risk adults at a work site near Stanford University (Meyer and Henderson, 1974). Approximately 30 hours of group instruction provided by dietitians and health educators over a 12-week period produced significant changes in the desired directions in dietary patterns (fewer fatty and cholesterol-rich foods consumed), blood cholesterol levels (lowered by an average of at least 17 mg/dl, depending on the treatment group), smoking (cut by 50% or more in all cases), and body weight (reduced by an average of at least 6.2 lb). About one-half of the sessions were devoted to nutrition education, including identification of health-promoting foods; guided practice in successive steps in new eating behaviors; reinforcement through peer approval; and progress monitoring. These methods were subsequently used in the Stanford Three-Community Study (Farquhar et al., 1977). Similarly, a simplified self-help kit to promote dietary change was pretested in families by the Stanford study investigators. Since the kit was successful in changing eating behaviors, the investigators then used the kit in the field in the subsequent Stanford Five-City Project (Elmore et al., 1982). The kit contained six lessons based on successive steps, beginning with a personal nutrition risk appraisal and then moving to specific shifts toward health-promoting food choices. This kit contained many other elements that have been effective in face-to-face group sessions, including methods to convey personal relevance, to monitor progress, and to obtain the involvement of family members.

To ensure that education is effective, its progress must be tracked through a *process evaluation*. Any activity such as health fairs, classes, contests, lectures, and point-of-purchase programs must be tracked and measures of its success must be obtained. Education provided through the mass media, including all forms of print, must similarly be tracked to ensure that the target audience is reached and that one's goals for education are reached. Process evaluations principally measure short-term success in achieving the conditions (such as attendance, satisfaction, attitudes, and knowledge) leading to behavior change (Farquhar, 1985a,b). Although these data will contribute to evaluating the overall outcome of the health education program, a complete outcome evaluation would require longer-term, more complete, and more rigorous methods. Nevertheless, process evaluation provides valuable information to the implementor on ways that educational programs and messages might be altered to improve their effectiveness in future applications.

Components and Amount of Nutrition Education Needed in Community-Based Programs

In the Stanford Three-Community Study and in the ongoing Stanford Five-City Project, investigators developed a general measure of the amount of education needed. Exposure to approximately 5 hours of education throughout the year provided both through the media and through occasional face-to-face encounters and continued for 2 or more years produced favorable change in all cardiovascular risk factors (e.g., blood cholesterol, blood pressure, smoking rate, exercise habits, and resting pulse rates) and more than a 20% reduction in saturated fat intake within the general population. Approximately 40% (or 2 hours) of this annual education was devoted to nutrition instruction designed principally to achieve attitude and behavior change. That experience suggests that if only 10% of the total exposure is devoted to face-to-face communication, the changes in diet observed (i.e., a greater than 20% reduction in saturated fat intake) can still occur (Farquhar et al., 1990). It is tempting to limit the face-to-face component of education to the least extent possible because of its cost. Its inclusion, however, is of great benefit for achieving and maintaining long-term dietary change. Additional experience in the Stanford Five-City Project derived from contests held at work sites and in the entire community indicates that incentives may help to maintain changes even in programs that rely largely on use of the media as the education method (King et al., 1987).

A person is more likely to adopt a new behavior if he or she is encouraged to do so through multiple channels, such as radio, television, print, point of purchase, small groups, schools, and work-site contests. For example, by taking advantage of the fact that parents often help their children with homework, a student's homework may be used to increase the parent's knowledge on nutrition and health. Coordinated programs with components that reinforce each other can be effective in reaching the most people (Farquhar et al., 1985a; King et al., 1987; Puska et al., 1981).

Successful maintenance of new dietary habits is dependent not only on *individual* factors such as knowledge, motivation, and skills but also on *system* factors, which comprise the physical and social environments of the individual. With individual factors, the nature of the health habit undergoing change has some relationship to maintenance. For example, weight changes, especially those resulting from periodic calorie restriction, are associated with rather high recidivism rates, whereas weight loss achieved through exercise is better maintained (King et al., 1989). Maintenance depends to a degree on the quality of the initial skills training program, e.g., its training in recidivism prevention skills, such as forewarning the participants of the social pressures that can precipitate a relapse. In addition, individuals who have changed their dietary habits through a phased approach that emphasizes the pleasure of new foods will often develop a new set of food preferences and then retain the new behaviors through internal motivation (Crouch et al., 1986; Fortmann et al., 1981; King et al., 1988; Meyer and Henderson, 1974).

The success of nutrition education in a group of people (e.g., students in a school, members of a community, or employees at a work site) is determined to a large extent by the initial proportion of that group who assimilated knowledge and changed behavior accordingly. The larger the proportion, the more likely that the newly adopted beneficial behavior will diffuse through the natural networks of the group (Rogers, 1983). Maintenance is thus partly dependent on the degree of initial success, but apparently, it also requires the adoption of health promotion activities by community organizations, including schools, hospitals, public health agencies, and citizens' groups, to supply ongoing reinforcement and reminders and to impart new knowledge and skills (Farquhar et al., 1985a, 1990).

The adoption and continued application of new technologies (such as use of principles of attitude change and social learning theory and the use of multiple channels of education) requires support from an organized structure of agencies and groups. For example, in order to ensure interorganizational collaboration, continuation could be supported by a nutrition council or nutrition consortium of all the organizations and individuals that impart nutrition knowledge and skills. An ongoing relationship between these community groups and external research and development organizations would ensure the dispersion of new technologies to promote behavior change as they become available.

In seeking comprehensive approaches that integrate various components (such as programs for schools or work sites or for point-of-purchase activities), it is necessary to identify all the subgroups within a population that require tailoring of nutrition education to their special needs. A successful program must take into consideration the characteristics of those who will receive the education. These include economic status, age, educational level, ethnic background, cultural values, health needs, health interest, and use of different media sources.

The three basic levels of communication should be explored: the network, the organization, and the community (see Table 3-3). Nutrition education, in its broadest sense, should encompass all subgroups reached through all three levels in order to achieve cost-effec-

TABLE 3-3 Sources of Health Communications

Network Level
Extended social networks
Peer groups
Families

Organization Level
Work sites
Restaurants
Grocery stores
Food producers and processors
Institutional food providers
Schools
Mass media organizations
Health-care organizations
Public health organizations
Government organizations

Community Level
Integrates network and organization levels, leading to change
in public opinion, social norms, legislation, food production, and
the social environment

---

tive and lasting change. This conclusion is based on the studies showing transitory effects in small groups, and on school or work-site programs conducted in isolation from broad, reinforcing community influences. The committee's review of these studies supports the common sense notion that change is more readily achieved if nutrition change programs include all three levels of communication.

It is clear from the studies discussed above that well-designed nutrition education programs are successful in a variety of settings and for a variety of people. Study results also demonstrate that unimaginative, information-only programs are not successful. The imagination of the learners must be captured; they must feel that the messages are personally relevant and that a stepwise course of action that avoids too much personal discomfort will yield tangible benefits (Bandura, 1986; Crouch et al., 1986; Killen et al., 1988; Meyer and Henderson, 1974).

Success requires both an adequate quantity and mix of effective instructional components. Appreciable changes in eating patterns have been maintained for 6 to 12 months in schools, work sites, and adult groups after approximately 7 to 15 hours of instruction given over a few months (Crouch et al., 1986; Killen et al., 1988; King et al., 1988; Meyer and Henderson, 1974). In addition, many people have improved their eating habits appreciably after being exposed to multifactor, comprehensive, community-based programs that included prolonged and intermittent exposure to approximately 2 hours of nutrition education per year for approximately 2 to 4 years (Farquhar et al., 1977, 1990).

Ingredients for success in both selected and general populations seem to require approximately equal proportions of (1) alerting, informing, and changing attitudes; (2) step-by-step active learning of self-directed behavior change methods; and (3) prevention of recidivism. Key elements of the first category include transmission of knowledge concerning diet-disease links and the provision of evidence of their relevance to the individual so that personal attitudes are changed. The learner must also gain knowledge of high-risk dietary patterns and of his or her own eating patterns. To accomplish this, the individual must learn monitoring methods, gain confidence from early successes, identify internal and external barriers to change, learn how to resist social pressures to change, and practice new skills in restaurant menu selection, label reading, food shopping, and food preparation and tasting. This effort is assisted by continued social support and maintenance incentives provided by others.

SUMMARY

The factors affecting food choices are numerous and complex. Some, such as inherent taste preferences and demographic trends, can be controlled little or not at all. Others more subject to modification include social norms, attitudes, skills, and availability of health-promoting foods. Over the past several decades, there have been important changes in food consumption patterns. Some of these changes are consistent with dietary recommendations (e.g., an increase in fish and vegetable consumption), but others are not (e.g., an increase in the consumption of high-fat ice cream). Similarly, recent changes in consumer attitudes and beliefs provide cause for both optimism and concern. Although there is a general trend toward recognition of the role of diet in disease prevention, surveys indicate that people are sometimes confused about which foods and food components are health-promoting and which are not.

Nevertheless, a review of current theory and practice with respect to attitude and behavior changes suggests that modification of food preferences and eating patterns is possible, but will require more than simply providing information to the population. People will need to be motivated to accept the information, see its personal relevance to them, integrate it into existing belief structures, acquire new skills and self-perceptions, and learn how to apply newly acquired attitudes to appropriate actions and to prevent recidivism. Various studies conducted within schools, at work sites, and in communities have indicated that intervention programs based on the communication/ persuasion model and the social learning model can be effective in producing substantial reductions in risk factors for diet-related diseases, particularly when they involve several components that reinforce each other and include the mass media. It seems very reasonable to infer from these studies that new national programs that implement favorable regulatory and food supply changes will enhance the impact of comprehensive education on the public's dietary patterns.

REFERENCES

Advertising Age. 1989. National ad spending by category. Advertising Age 60:8.

Ajzen, I. 1989. Attitudes, Personality, and Behavior. Wadsworth, Florence, Ky. 150 pp.

Ajzen, I., and M. Fishbein. 1980. Understanding Attitudes and Predicting Social Behavior. Prentice-Hall, Englewood Cliffs, N.J. 278 pp.

Arntzenius, A.C., D. Kromhout, J.D. Barth, J.H.C. Reiber, A.V.G. Bruschke, B. Buis, C.M. van Gent, N. Kempen-Voogd, S. Strikwerda, and E.A. van der Velde. 1985. Diet, lipoproteins, and the progression of coronary atherosclerosis: the Leiden Intervention Trial. N. Engl. J. Med. 312:805-811.

Atkin, C.K. 1979. Research evidence on mass mediated health communication campaigns. Pp. 655-668 in D. Nimmo, ed. Communication Yearbook 3. Transaction Books, New Brunswick, N.J.

Axelson, M.L., T.L. Federline, and D. Brinberg. 1985. A meta-analysis of food- and nutrition-related research. J. Nutr. Educ. 17:51-54.

Bandura, A. 1977. Social Learning Theory. Prentice-Hall, Englewood Cliffs, N.J. 247 pp.

Bandura, A. 1982. Self-efficacy mechanism in human agency. Am. Psychol. 37:122-147.

Bandura, A. 1986. Social Foundations of Thought and Action: a Social Cognitive Theory. Prentice-Hall, Englewood Cliffs, N.J. 617 pp.

Beauchamp, G.K., and M. Moran. 1982. Dietary experience and sweet taste preference in human infants. Appetite 3:139-152.

Belasco, W.J. 1989. Appetite for Change: How the Counterculture Took on the Food Industry, 1966-1988. Pantheon Books, New York. 311 pp.

Best, J.A. 1989. Intervention perspectives on school health promotion research. Health Educ. Q. 16:299-306.

Best, J.A., S.J. Thomson, S.M. Santi, E.A. Smith, and K.S. Brown. 1988. Preventing cigarette smoking among school children. Annu. Rev. Public Health 9:161-201.

Birch, L.L. 1987. The acquisition of food acceptance patterns in children. Pp. 107-130 in R.A. Boakes, D.A. Popplewell, and M.J. Burton, eds. Eating Habits: Food, Physiology, and Learned Behavior. John Wiley & Sons, Chichester, Great Britain.

Blackburn, H., R. Luepker, F.G. Kline, N. Bracht, R. Carlaw, D. Jacobs, M. Mittelmark, L. Stauffer, and H.L. Taylor. 1984. The Minnesota Heart Health Program: a research and demonstration project in cardiovascular disease prevention. Pp. 1171-1178 in J.D. Matarazzo, S.M. Weiss, J.A. Herd, N.E. Miller, and S.M. Weiss, eds. Behavioral Health: A Handbook of Health Enhancement and Disease Prevention. John Wiley & Sons, New York.

Blair, S.N., P.V. Piserchia, C.S. Wilbur, and J.H. Crowder. 1986. A public health intervention model for work-site health promotion: impact on exercise and physical fitness in a health promotion plan after 24 months. J. Am. Med. Assoc. 255:921-926.

Bogart, L. 1967. Strategy in Advertising. Harcourt, Brace, & World, New York. 336 pp.

Bruno, R., C. Arnold, L. Jacobson, M. Winick, and E. Wynder. 1983. Randomized controlled trial of a nonpharmacologic cholesterol reduction program at the worksite. Prev. Med. 12:523-532.

Burros, M. January 6, 1988. What Americans really eat: nutrition can wait. New York Times. C1, C6.

Calorie Control Council. 1989. 1989 National Survey. Conducted by Booth Research Services for the Calorie Control Council, Atlanta, Ga. Various pagings.

Capps, O., Jr. 1986. Changes in domestic demand for food: impacts on Southern agriculture. South. J. Agric. Econ. 18:25-36.

Carmody, T.P., S.G. Fey, D.K. Pierce, W.E. Connor, and J.D. Matarazzo. 1982. Behavioral treatment of hyperlipidemia: techniques, results, and future directions. J. Behav. Med. 5:91-96.

Carmody, T.P., J. Istvan, J.D. Matarazzo, S.L. Connor, and W.E. Connor. 1986. Applications of social learning theory in the promotion of heart-healthy diets: the Family Heart Study intervention model. Health Educ. Res. 1:13-27.

Chaiken, S. 1987. The heuristic model of persuasion. Pp. 3-39 in M.P. Zanna, J.M. Olson, and C.P. Herman, eds. Social Influence: the Ontario Symposium. Vol. 5. Lawrence Erlbaum Associates, Hillsdale, N.J.

Chaiken, S., and C. Stangor. 1987. Attitudes and attitude change. Annu. Rev. Psychol. 38:575-630.

Cialdini, R.B., R.E. Petty, and J.T. Cacioppo. 1981. Attitude and attitude change. Annu. Rev. Psychol. 32:357-404.

Contento, I.R., J.L. Michela, and C.J. Goldberg. 1988. Food choice among adolescents: population segmentation by motivations. J. Nutr. Educ. 20:289-298.

Cooper, J., and R.T. Croyle. 1984. Attitudes and attitude change. Annu. Rev. Psychol. 35:395-426.

Crouch, M., J.F. Sallis, J.W. Farquhar, W.L. Haskell, N.M. Ellsworth, A.B. King, and T. Rogers. 1986. Personal and mediated health counseling for sustained dietary reduction of hypercholesterolemia. Prev. Med. 15:282-291.

Davis, C.M. 1928. Self selection of diet by newly weaned infants: an experimental study. Am. J. Dis. Child. 36:651-679.

Davis, C.M. 1934. Studies in the self-selection of diet by young children. J. Am. Dent. Assoc. 21:636-640.

Desor, J.A., O. Maller, and L.S. Greene. 1977. Preference for sweet in humans: infants, children, and adults. Pp. 161-172 in J.M. Weiffenbach, ed. Taste and Development: the Genesis of Sweet Preference. DHEW Publ. No. (NIH) 77-1068. National Institutes of Health, Public Health Service, U.S. Department of Health, Education, and Welfare, Bethesda, Md.

DHHS (U.S. Department of Health and Human Services). 1988. The Surgeon General's Report on Nutrition and Health. DHHS (PHS) Publ. No. 88-50210. Public Health

Service, U.S. Department of Health and Human Services. U.S. Government Printing Office, Washington, D.C. 727 pp.

Drewnowski, A., J.D. Brunzell, K. Sande, P.H. Iverius, and M.R.C. Greenwood. 1985. Sweet tooth reconsidered: taste responsiveness in human obesity. Physiol. Behav. 35:617-622.

Duewer, L.A. 1989. Changes in the beef and pork industries. Natl. Food Rev. 12(1):5-8.

Dugas, C. 1985. Countermarketing: "bad" foods fight back. Ad Forum 6:18-22.

Egger, G., W. Fitzgerald, G. Frape, A. Monaem, P. Rubinstein, C. Tyler, and B. McKay. 1983. Results of a large scale media antismoking campaign in Australia: North Coast "Quit For Life" programme. Br. Med. J. 287:1125-1128.

Ehnholm, C., J.K. Huttunen, P. Pietinen, U. Leino, M. Mutanen, E. Kostiainen, J. Pikkarainen, R. Dougherty, J. Iacono, and P. Puska. 1982. Effect of diet on serum lipoproteins in a population with a high risk of coronary heart disease. N. Engl. J. Med. 307:850-855.

Ellison, R.C., A.L. Capper, R.J. Goldberg, J.C. Witschi, and F.J. Stare. 1989. Changing school food services to promote cardiovascular health. Health Educ. Q. 16:171-180.

Elmore, J., C.B. Taylor, and J.A. Flora. 1982. Self-help nutrition kit with a nutrition booklet. Internal formative research report prepared for the Stanford Heart Disease Prevention Program. Stanford, Calif.

Erickson, J.L. 1989. Simplot bites back in micro snack war. Advertising Age 60:4.

Fabsitz, R., M. Feinleib, and Z. Hrubec. 1980. Weight changes in adult twins. Acta Genet. Med. Gemellol. 29:273-279.

Falciglia, G.A., and J.D. Gussow. 1980. Television commercials and eating behavior of obese and normal-weight women. J. Nutr. Educ. 12:196-199.

Farb, P., and G. Armelagos. 1980. Consuming Passions: the Anthropology of Eating. Houghton Mifflin, Boston. 279 pp.

Farquhar, J.W., N. Maccoby, P.D. Wood, J.K. Alexander, H. Breitrose, B.W. Brown, Jr., W.L. Haskell, A.L. McAlister, A.J. Meyer, J.D. Nash, and M.P. Stern. 1977. Community education for cardiovascular health. Lancet 1:1192-1195.

Farquhar, J.W., N. Maccoby, and P.D. Wood. 1985a. Education and communication studies. Pp. 207-221 in W.W. Holland, R. Detels, and G. Knox, eds. Oxford Textbook of Public Health. Vol. 3. Investigative Methods in Public Health. Oxford University Press, London.

Farquhar, J.W., S.P. Fortmann, N. Maccoby, W.L. Haskell, P.T. Williams, J.A. Flora, C.B. Taylor, B.W. Brown, Jr., D.S. Solomon, and S.B. Hulley. 1985b. The Stanford Five-City Project: design and methods. Am. J. Epidemiol. 122:323-334.

Farquhar, J.W., S.P. Fortmann, J.A. Flora, C.B. Taylor, W.L. Haskell, P.T. Williams, N. Maccoby, and P.D. Wood. 1990. Effects of communitywide education on cardiovascular disease risk factors. J. Am. Med. Assoc. 264:359-365.

Fazio, R.H. 1990. Multiple processes by which attitudes guide behavior: the MODE model as an integrative framework. Pp. 75-109 in M. Zanna, ed. Advances in Experimental Social Psychology. Academic Press, New York.

Fazio, R.H., and M.P. Zanna. 1981. Direct experience and attitude-behavior consistency. Adv. Exp. Soc. Psychol. 14:161-202.

Fletcher, H. 1899. Nature's Food Filter or What and When To Swallow. Herbert S. Stone & Company, Chicago. 29 pp.

FMI (Food Marketing Institute). 1989. Trends: Consumer Attitudes & the Supermarket, 1989. Conducted for Food Marketing Institute by Opinion Research Corporation. The Research Department, Food Marketing Institute, Washington, D.C. 65 pp.

FMI (Food Marketing Institute). 1990. Trends: Consumer Attitudes & the Supermarket, 1990. Conducted for Food Marketing Institute by Opinion Research Corporation. The Research Department, Food Marketing Institute, Washington, D.C. 70 pp.

Fortmann, S.P., P.T. Williams, S.B. Hulley, W.L Haskell, and J.W. Farquhar. 1981. Effect of health education on dietary behavior: the Stanford Three Community Study. Am. J. Clin. Nutr. 34:2030-2038.

Freimuth, V.S. 1990. The chronically uninformed: closing the knowledge gap in health. Pp. 171-186 in E.B. Ray and L. Donohew, eds. Communication and Health: Systems and Applications. Lawrence Erlbaum Associates, Hillsdale, N.J.

Freimuth, V.S., and W. Mettger. 1990. Is there a hard-to-reach audience? Public Health Rep. 105:232-238.

Freimuth, V.S., S.L. Hammond, and J.A. Stein. 1988. Health advertising: prevention for profit. Am. J. Public Health 78:557-561.

Garb, J.L., and A.J. Stunkard. 1974. Taste aversions in man. Am. J. Psychiatr. 131:1204-1207.

Glanz, K. 1985. Nutrition education for risk factor reduction and patient education: a review. Prev. Med. 14:721-752.

Glanz, K., and R.M. Mullis. 1988. Environmental interventions to promote healthy eating: a review of models, programs, and evidence. Health Educ. Q. 15:395-415.

Glanz, K., and T. Seewald-Klein. 1986. Nutrition at the worksite: an overview. J. Nutr. Educ. 18:S1-S12.

Goldberg, M.E., and J. Hartwick. 1990. The effects of advertiser reputation and extremity of advertising claim on product evaluation. J. Consumer Res. 17:185-192.

Green, L.W. 1975. Diffusion and adoption of innovations related to cardiovascular risk behavior in the public. Pp. 84-108 in A.J. Enelow and J.B. Henderson, eds. Applying Behavioral Science to Cardiovascular Risk: Proceedings of a Conference. American Heart Association, Dallas, Tex.

Greene, C. 1988. A new look for supermarket produce sections. Natl. Food Rev. 11(4):1-5.

Gutzwiller, F., B. Nater, and J. Martin. 1985. Community-based primary prevention of cardiovascular disease in Switzerland: methods and results of the National Research Program (NRP 1A). Prev. Med. 14:482-491.

Harris, M. 1985. Good To Eat: Riddles of Food and Culture. Simon and Schuster, New York. 289 pp.

Hewitt, L.E., and H.T. Blaine. 1984. Prevention through mass media communication. Pp. 281-326 in P.M. Miller and T.D. Nirenberg, eds. Prevention of Alcohol Abuse. Plenum Press, New York.

Hjermann, I., K.V. Byre, I. Holme, and P. Leren. 1981. Effect of diet and smoking intervention on the incidence of coronary heart disease. Lancet 2:1303-1310.

Janz, N.K., and M.H. Becker. 1984. The Health Belief Model: a decade later. Health Educ. Q. 11:1-47.

Ketchum Communications. 1989. The Potato Board: How To Give a Greatly Misunderstood Food a Fresh Perception. Ketchum Communications, San Francisco, Calif. 1 p.

Killen, J.D. 1985. Prevention of adolescent tobacco smoking: the social pressure resistance training approach. J. Child. Psychol. Psychiatr. 26:7-15.

Killen, J.D., M.J. Telch, T.N. Robinson, N. Maccoby, C.B. Taylor, and J.W. Farquhar. 1988. Cardiovascular disease risk reduction for tenth graders: a multiple-factor school-based approach. J. Am. Med. Assoc. 260:1728-1733.

King, A.C., J.A. Flora, S.P. Fortmann, and C.B. Taylor. 1987. Smokers' challenge: immediate and long-term findings of a community smoking cessation contest. Am. J. Public Health 77:1340-1341.

King, A.C., K.E. Saylor, S. Foster, J.D. Killen, M.J. Telch, J.W. Farquhar, and J.A. Flora.

1988. Promoting dietary change in adolescents: a school-based approach for modifying and maintaining healthful behavior. Am. J. Prev. Med. 4:68-74.

King, A.C., B. Frey-Hewitt, D.M. Dreon, and P.D. Wood. 1989. Diet vs. exercise in weight maintenance. Arch. Intern. Med. 149:2741-2746.

Kinsey, J. 1983. Working wives and the marginal propensity to consume food away from home. Am. J. Agric. Econ. 65:10-19.

Klesges, R.C., M.M. Vasey, and R.E. Glasgow. 1986. A worksite smoking modification competition: potential for public health impact. Am. J. Public Health 76:198-200.

Kotler, P., and G. Zaltmann. 1971. Social marketing: an approach to planned social change. J. Market. 35:3-12.

Kreuter, M.W., G.M. Christenson, and R. Davis. 1984. School health education research: future issues and challenges. J. School Health 54:27-32.

Lantis, M. 1962. The child consumer: cultural. J. Home Econ. 54:570-579.

Lasater, T., D. Abrams, L. Artz, P. Beaudin, L. Cabrera, J. Elder, A. Ferreira, P. Knisley, G. Peterson, A. Rodrigues, P. Rosenberg, R. Snow, and R. Carleton. 1984. Lay volunteer delivery of a community-based cardiovascular risk factor change program: the Pawtucket Experiment. Pp. 1166-1170 in J.D. Matarazzo, S.M. Weiss, J.A. Herd, N.E. Miller, and S.M. Weiss, eds. Behavioral Health: A Handbook of Health Enhancement and Disease Prevention. John Wiley & Sons, New York.

Lefebvre, R.C., and J.A. Flora. 1988. Social marketing and public health intervention. Health Educ. Q. 15:299-315.

Levy, A.S., and R.C. Stokes. 1987. Effects of a health promotion advertising campaign on sales of ready-to-eat cereals. Public Health Rep. 102:398-403.

Levy, A.S., N. Ostrove, T. Guthrie, and J.T. Heimbach. 1988. Recent Trends and Beliefs about Diet/Disease Relationships: Results of the 1979-1988 FDA Health and Diet Surveys. Presented at FDA/USDA Food Editors Conference: December 1-2, 1988. Division of Consumer Studies, Center for Food Safety and Applied Nutrition, Food and Drug Administration, U.S. Department of Health and Human Services, Washington, D.C.

Lewin, K. 1943. Forces behind food habits and methods of change. Pp. 35-65 in The Problem of Changing Food Habits. Report of the Committee on Food Habits 1941-1943. Bulletin of the National Research Council, No. 108. National Academy of Sciences, Washington, D.C.

Light, L., J. Tenney, B. Portnoy, L. Kessler, A.B. Rodgers, B. Patterson, O. Mathews, E. Katz, J.E. Blair, S.K. Evans, and E. Tuckermanty. 1989. Eat for Health: a nutrition and cancer control supermarket intervention. Public Health Rep. 104:443-450.

Maccoby, N., J.W. Farquhar, P.D. Wood, and J. Alexander. 1977. Reducing the risk of cardiovascular disease: effects of a community-based campaign on knowledge and behavior. J. Community Health 3:100-114.

Manoff, R.K. 1985. Social Marketing: New Imperative for Public Health. Praeger, New York. 293 pp.

Marshall, J.F. 1971. Topics and networks in intra-village communication. Pp. 160-166 in S. Polgar, ed. Culture and Population: a Collection of Current Studies. Schenkman Publishing, Cambridge, Mass.

Mayer, J. 1968. Overweight: Causes, Cost, and Control. Prentice-Hall, Englewood Cliffs, N.J. 213 pp.

McGuire, W.J. 1964. Inducing resistance to persuasion: some contemporary approaches. Adv. Exp. Soc. Psychol. 1:191-229.

McGuire, W.J. 1985. Attitudes and attitude change. Pp. 233-346 in G. Lindzey and E. Aronson, eds. Handbook of Social Psychology, 3rd ed. Vol. II. Random House, New York.

McGuire, W.J. 1989. Theoretical foundations of campaigns. Pp. 39-42 in R.E. Rice and C.K. Atkin, eds. Public Communication Campaigns, 2nd ed. Sage, Newbury Park, Calif.

McGuire, W.J., and D. Papageorgis. 1961. The relative efficacy of various types of prior belief-defense in producing immunity against persuasion. J. Abnorm. Soc. Psychol. 62:327-337.

Meyer, A.J., and J.B. Henderson. 1974. Multiple risk factor reduction in the prevention of cardiovascular disease. Prev. Med. 3:225-236.

Meyer, A.J., N. Maccoby, and J.W. Farquhar. 1977. The role of opinion leadership in a cardiovascular health education campaign. Pp. 579-591 in B.D. Ruben, ed. Communication Yearbook 1. Transaction Books, New Brunswick, N.J.

Michela, J.L., and I.R. Contento. 1984. Spontaneous classification of foods by elementary school-aged children. Health Educ. Q. 11:57-76.

Michela, J.L., and I.R. Contento. 1986. Cognitive, motivational, social, and environmental influences on children's food choices. Health Psychol. 5:209-230.

Miller, N., E. Wagner, and P. Rogers. 1988. Worksite-based multifactorial risk intervention trial. J. Am. Coll. Cardiol. 11:207A.

Montagu, M.F.A. 1962. Prenatal Influences. Charles C Thomas, Springfield, Ill. 614 pp.

Moskowitz, H.W., H.L. Jacobs, and S.D. Sharma. 1975. Cross-cultural differences in simple taste preferences. Science 190:1217-1218.

Mothner, I. 1987. Our national food fight. We're eating lots of fruits and veggies, but more fats, snacks and sweets, too. Am. Health 6:48-49.

MRFIT Research Group. 1982. Multiple Risk Factor Intervention Trial: risk factor changes and mortality results. J. Am. Med. Assoc. 248:1465-1477.

Mullis, R.M., and P. Pirie. 1988. Lean meats make the grade—a collaborative nutrition intervention program. J. Am. Diet. Assoc. 88:191-195.

Mullis, R.M., M.K. Hunt, M. Foster, L. Hachfeld, D. Lansing, P. Snyder, and P. Pirie. 1987. The Shop Smart for Your Heart grocery program. J. Nutr. Educ. 19:225-228.

Nader, P.R., J.F. Sallis, J. Rupp, C. Atkins, T. Patterson, and I. Abramson. 1986. San Diego family health project: reaching families through the schools. J. School Health 56:227-231.

Nickens, H.W. 1990. Commentary: health promotion and disease prevention among minorities. Health Affairs 9:133-143.

NRC (National Research Council). 1989. Diet and Health: Implications for Reducing Chronic Disease Risk. Report of the Committee on Diet and Health, Food and Nutrition Board, Commission on Life Sciences. National Academy Press, Washington, D.C. 749 pp.

Perry, C.L., R.V. Luepker, D.M. Murray, M.D. Hearn, A. Halper, B. Dudovitz, M.C. Maile, and M. Smyth. 1989. Parent involvement with children's health promotion: a one year follow-up of the Minnesota home team. Health Educ. Q. 16:171-180.

Petty, R.E., and J.T. Cacioppo. 1981. Attitudes and Persuasion: Classic and Contemporary Approaches. W.C. Brown, Dubuque, Iowa. 314 pp.

Petty, R.E., and J.T. Cacioppo. 1984. Motivational factors in consumer response to advertisements. Pp. 418-454 in R.G. Geen, W.W. Beatty, and R.M. Arkin, eds. Human Motivation: Physiological, Behavioral, and Social Approaches. Allyn and Bacon, New York.

Petty, R.E., and J.T. Cacioppo. 1986. Communication and Persuasion: Central and Peripheral Routes to Attitude Change. Springer-Verlag, New York. 262 pp.

Popkin, B.M., P.S. Haines, and K.C. Reidy. 1989. Food consumption trends of US women: patterns and determinants between 1977 and 1985. Am. J. Clin. Nutr. 49:1307-1319.

Progressive Grocer. 1986. The cream also rises. Record growth for the ice cream business is being fueled by two new scoops: superpremiums and frozen novelties. Progressive Grocer 65:115.

Puska, P. 1985. Effectiveness of nutrition intervention strategies. Pp. 39-46 in E.M.E. van den Berg, W. Bosman, and B.C. Breedveld, eds. Nutrition in Europe: Proceedings of the Fourth European Nutrition Conference. Voorlichtingsbureau voor de Voeding, The Hague, The Netherlands.

Puska, P., K. Koskela, A. McAlister, U. Pallonen, E. Vartiainen, and K. Homan. 1979. A comprehensive television smoking cessation program in Finland. Int. J. Health Educ. Suppl. 22:1-28.

Puska, P., J. Tuomilehto, J. Salonen, A. Nissinen, J. Virtamo, S. Björkqvist, K. Koskela, L. Neittaanmäki, L. Takalo, T.E. Kottke, J. Mäki, P. Sipilä, and P. Varvikko. 1981. Community Control of Cardiovascular Diseases: the North Karelia Project. World Health Organization, Copenhagen, Denmark. 351 pp.

Puska, P., K. Koskela, A. McAlister, H. Mäyränen, A. Smolander, S. Moisio, L. Viri, V. Korpelainen, and E.M. Rogers. 1986. Use of lay opinion leaders to promote diffusion of health innovations in a community programme: lessons learned from the North Karelia project. Bull. W.H.O. 64:437-446.

Putnam, J.J. 1989. Food Consumption, Prices, and Expenditures, 1966-87. Statistical Bulletin No. 773. Economic Research Service, U.S. Department of Agriculture, Washington, D.C. 111 pp.

Ravussin, E., S. Lillioja, W.C. Knowler, L. Christin, D. Freymond, W.G. Abbott, V. Boyce, B.V. Howard, and C. Bogardus. 1988. Reduced rate of energy expenditure as a risk factor for body-weight gain. N. Engl. J. Med. 318:467-472.

Roberts, D.F., and N. Maccoby. 1985. Effects of mass communication. Pp. 539-598 in G. Lindzey and E. Aronson, eds. Handbook of Social Psychology, 3rd ed. Vol. II. Random House, New York.

Roberts, S.B., J. Savage, W.A. Coward, B. Chew, and A. Lucas. 1988. Energy expenditure and intake in infants born to lean and overweight mothers. N. Engl. J. Med. 318:461-466.

Rodin, J. 1980. Social and immediate environmental influences on food selection. Int. J. Obesity 4:364-370.

Rogers, E.M. 1983. Diffusion of Innovations, 3rd ed. Free Press, New York. 453 pp.

Rootman, I. 1985. Using health promotion to reduce alcohol problems. Pp. 57-81 in M. Grant, ed. Alcohol Policies. WHO Regional Publications, European Series No. 18. World Health Organization, Copenhagen, Denmark.

Rosenstock, I.M. 1974. Historical origins of the Health Belief Model. Health Educ. Monogr. 2:328-335.

Rosenstock, I.M., V.J. Strecher, and M.H. Becker. 1988. Social learning theory and the Health Belief Model. Health Educ. Q. 15:175-183.

Rossouw, J.E., P.L. Jooste, J.P. Kotze, and P.C.J. Jordaan. 1981. The control of hypertension in two communities: an interim evaluation. S. Afr. Med. J. 60:208-212.

Rozin, P., and D. Schiller. 1980. The nature and acquisition of a preference of chili pepper by humans. Motiv. Emotion 4:77-101.

Sallis, J.F., R.D. Hill, S.P. Fortmann, and J.A. Flora. 1986. Health behavior change at the worksite: cardiovascular risk reduction. Prog. Behav. Modif. 20:161-197.

Schoenborn, C.A., and B.H. Cohen. 1986. Trends in Smoking, Alcohol Consumption and Other Health Practices Among U.S. Adults, 1977 and 1983. NCHS Advance Data from Vital & Health Statistics, No. 118. National Center for Health Statistics, Public Health Service, U.S. Department of Health and Human Services, Hyattsville, Md. 13 pp.

Sclafani, A., and D. Springer. 1976. Dietary obesity in adult rats: similarities to hypo-
thalamic and human obesity syndromes. Physiol. Behav. 17:461-471.

Senauer, B. 1986. Economics and nutrition. Pp. 46-57 in What Is America Eating?
Proceedings of a Symposium. Food and Nutrition Board, Commission on Life
Sciences. National Academy Press, Washington, D.C.

Sheppard, B.H., J. Hartwick, and P.R. Warshaw. 1988. The theory of reasoned action:
a meta-analysis of past research with recommendations for modifications and future
research. J. Consumer Res. 15:325-343.

Sherman, S.J. 1987. Cognitive processes in the formation, change, and expression of
attitudes. Pp. 75-106 in M.P. Zanna, J.M. Olson, and C.P. Herman, eds. Social
Influence: the Ontario Symposium. Vol. 5. Lawrence Erlbaum Associates, Hillsdale,
N.J.

Smallwood, D., and J. Blaylock. 1981. Impact of Household Size and Income on Food
Spending Patterns. Technical Bulletin No. 1650. National Economics Division,
Economics and Statistics Service, U.S. Department of Agriculture, Washington, D.C.
22 pp.

Smith, K. 1990. Alar: One Year Later. A Media Analysis of a Hypothetical Health
Risk. American Council on Science and Health, New York. 10 pp.

Staats, A.W., and C.K. Staats. 1958. Attitudes established by classical conditioning. J.
Abnorm. Soc. Psychol. 57:37-40.

Steiner, J.E. 1977. Facial expressions of the neonate infant indicating the hedonics of
food-related chemical stimuli. Pp. 173-190 in J.M. Weiffenbach, ed. Taste and
Development: the Genesis of the Sweet Preference. DHEW Publ. No. (NIH) 77-
1068. National Institutes of Health, Public Health Service, U.S. Department of Health,
Education, and Welfare, Bethesda, Md.

Stone, E. 1985. School-based health research funded by the National Heart, Lung, and
Blood Institute. J. School Health 55:168-174.

Stone, E.J., C.L. Perry, and R.V. Leupker. 1989. Synthesis of cardiovascular behavioral
research for youth health promotion. Health Educ. Q. 16:155-169.

Strong, E.K. 1925. The Psychology of Selling and Advertising. McGraw-Hill, New
York. 468 pp.

Stunkard, A.J., M.R.J. Felix, and R.Y. Cohen. 1985. Mobilizing a community to promote
health: the Pennsylvania County Health Improvement Program (CHIP). Pp. 143-190
in J.C. Rosen and L.J. Solomon, eds. Prevention in Health Psychology. University
Press of New England, Hanover.

Supermarket Business. 1986. 39th Annual Consumer Expenditures Study. Americans
as artifacts: examining today's shoppers through their spending habits. Supermarket
Business. September, pp. 69, 88.

Szalai, A. 1972. The Use of Time: Daily Activities of Urban and Suburban Populations
in Twelve Countries. Mouton Press, The Hague, The Netherlands. 868 pp.

Telch, M.J., J.D. Killen, A.L. McAlister, C.L. Perry, and N. Maccoby. 1982. Long-term
follow-up of a pilot project on smoking prevention with adolescents. J. Behav.
Med. 5:1-8.

Tuomilehto, J., J. Geboers, J.T. Salonen, A. Nissinen, K. Kuulasmaa, and P. Puska.
1986. Decline in cardiovascular mortality in North Karelia and other parts of Finland. Br. Med. J. 293:1068-1071.

U.S. Department of Commerce. 1983. Statistical Abstract of the United States, 1982-83,
103rd ed. Bureau of the Census, U.S. Department of Commerce. U.S. Government
Printing Office, Washington, D.C. 1042 pp.

USDA (U.S. Department of Agriculture). 1953. Consumption of Food in the United
States, 1902-1952. Agriculture Handbook No. 62. Bureau of Agricultural Economics, U.S. Department of Agriculture, Washington, D.C. 249 pp.

USDA (U.S. Department of Agriculture). 1985. Nationwide Food Consumption Survey Continuing Survey of Food Intakes by Individuals: Women 19-50 Years and Their Children 1-5 Years, 1 Day, 1985. Report No. 85-1. Nutrition Monitoring Division, Human Nutrition Information Service, U.S. Department of Agriculture, Washington, D.C. 102 pp.

USDA (U.S. Department of Agriculture). 1989. Table on production and per capita consumption of soft drinks and soft drinks by flavor. Economic Research Service, U.S. Department of Agriculture, Washington, D.C. 2 pp.

Weiffenbach, J.M. 1977. Sensory mechanisms in the newborn's tongue. Pp. 205-213 in J.M. Weiffenbach, ed. Taste and Development: the Genesis of the Sweet Preference. DHEW Publ. No. (NIH) 77-1068. National Institutes of Health, Public Health Service, U.S. Department of Health, Education, and Welfare, Bethesda, Md.

White, S.L., and S.K. Maloney. 1990. Promoting healthy diets and active lives to heard-to-reach groups: market research study. Public Health Rep. 105:224-231.

WHO (World Health Organization). 1986. Community Prevention and Control of Cardiovascular Diseases. Technical Report Series No. 732. Report of a WHO Expert Committee. World Health Organization, Geneva, Switzerland. 62 pp.

Wilbur, C.S. 1983. The Johnson & Johnson Program. Prev. Med. 12:672-681.

Wilhelmsen, L., G. Berglund, D. Elmfeldt, G. Tibblin, H. Wedel, K. Pennert, A. Vedin, C. Wilhelmsson, and L. Werkö. 1986. The multifactor primary prevention trial in Göteborg, Sweden. Eur. Heart J. 7:279-288.

Woteki, C.E. 1986. Methods for surveying food habits: how do we know what Americans are eating? Clin. Nutr. 5:9-16.

Yankelovich, Skelly and White, Inc. 1985. Consumer Climate for Meat Products. Prepared for the American Meat Institute, Washington, D.C., and the National Live Stock and Meat Board, Chicago, Ill.

4

Interpretation and Application of the Recommendations in the *Diet and Health* Report

EFFECTIVE IMPLEMENTATION of dietary recommendations requires, at a minimum, that they be interpreted in a consistent manner and have broad applicability. In this chapter, the committee interprets the recommendations in the Food and Nutrition Board's *Diet and Health* report (NRC, 1989a) and describes how implementors in all sectors of society can use them to teach consumers how to improve their diets. However, this discussion is designed to be applicable to most sets of dietary recommendations and guidelines prepared by various expert bodies.

INTERPRETATION OF THE *DIET AND HEALTH* RECOMMENDATIONS

The *Diet and Health* recommendations pertain to every healthy North American from age 2. Quantitative target levels in the recommendations were based on expert judgment as to whether these levels are likely to be attained by the population. The Committee on Diet and Health believed its recommendations could be achieved without drastic changes in usual dietary patterns and without undue risk of nutrient deficiencies. This committee agrees with that view. People with medical problems and those on special diets should seek professional advice on the applicability of the recommendations to them. Infants and children under age 2 have special dietary needs that are not covered by dietary recommendations; expert advice on their nutritional needs can be obtained from pediatricians or nutritionists who work with these groups.

84

A person's entire dietary pattern, rather than individual meals or snacks, should be planned to meet the recommendations. The Committee on Diet and Health did not specify the period during which one's dietary pattern should meet these goals (e.g., over the course of a day or a week) but implied that routine eating patterns should be compatible with them. The extensive data base from which they were derived indicates that the risk of several chronic diseases is likely to be reduced among populations whose routine dietary patterns are similar to those advocated by that committee. To move toward such an eating pattern, this committee believes that consumers should plan their *daily* diet to achieve it, but that flexibility should predominate over rigid self-discipline. For example, people should not be alarmed if their diets on any given day do not fully or precisely meet the recommendations. In general, menu planning is simplified when it is focused on a day, several days, or a week rather than single meals as time frames during which the recommendations should be met.

The *Diet and Health* recommendations were presented in a logical sequence that also reflected a general order of importance. Highest priority is given to reducing fat intake, since the scientific evidence linking dietary fats and other lipids to health is strongest and the likely impact from dietary change on public health is the greatest. Lower priority was given to recommendations on other dietary components because they are derived from weaker evidence or because their public health impact is not likely to be as strong. The Committee on Diet and Health emphasized, however, that maximum benefits to health are likely to be achieved by basing meal patterns on all nine recommendations and the Recommended Dietary Allowances (RDAs) (NRC, 1989b).

Thus, efforts to implement dietary recommendations should focus primarily on encouraging and teaching people to limit their consumption of total fat, saturated fat, and cholesterol. As people modify their diets to meet this most important recommendation, they should find little difficulty in meeting the next two recommendations—to increase intake of carbohydrates and to limit protein intake. The best way to reduce fat intake is to eat more low-fat foods, such as grains, vegetables, legumes, and fruits (thereby eating more carbohydrates) and, if desired, moderate portions of meat, poultry, and fish (thereby limiting protein intake). Nutrient adequacy, the focus of several other recommendations, is likely to be achieved by the judicious selection of a plant-enriched diet containing some lean meats and low-fat dairy products. The Committee on Diet and Health emphasized that, depending on need, the calories lost by reducing dietary fat intake should be made up by consuming carbohydrate-rich plant foods such as cereals, fruits, and vegetables rather than high-protein foods. Most people in the United States consume more than enough protein, as is discussed later in this chapter.

The *Diet and Health* recommendations can be followed by people who consume almost any culturally, ethnically, or regionally specific cuisine, since they encourage the use of a wide variety of foods. They are especially suitable for many ethnic cuisines (e.g., Chinese and Indian) that tend to be lower in total fat, saturated fat, and cholesterol and higher in plant foods and complex carbohydrates than traditional Western cuisines. Nevertheless, such cuisines may need to be modified (e.g., less sodium-rich soy sauce in Chinese cooking).

Lack of access to a wide variety of nutritionally desirable foods is a formidable barrier to eating well, especially for people on limited incomes who must shop in stores with limited choices. It may not be possible, for example, for such people to drink low-fat or skim milk if local food stores charge premium prices for them or stock only whole milk. Dietary recommendations can be followed by those on limited incomes if they shop carefully at stores with an adequate selection of foods and reasonable prices. In selecting meat, poultry, and fish, less expensive cuts should be chosen; legumes (dried beans and peas) should be used in place of these foods as necessary or desired. Grain products are relatively inexpensive, as are many fresh vegetables and fruits in season or frozen or canned produce. Low-fat and skim milk and low- or nonfat dairy products often cost less than whole milk and products made from it.

The Committee on Diet and Health advocated the consumption of a wide variety of foods; it did not prohibit specific foods or food products, since the nutritional composition of the total diet is of most importance. Nevertheless, consumers will need to limit their consumption of oils, fats, egg yolks, and salt as well as fried and other fatty foods. For example, it would not be possible to limit cholesterol intake to less than 300 mg/day without limiting egg yolks to an average of one or less daily.

The RDAs provide sex- and age-specific guidelines on the levels of intake of essential nutrients judged to be adequate to meet the needs of most healthy people. Although they are set high enough to exceed the nutrient requirements of most people, it is difficult to determine the needs of any individual. Therefore, it is prudent to recommend that consumers eat diets that provide nutrients at approximate RDA levels. Consumers are likely to meet the *Diet and Health* recommendations and the RDAs if they consume adequate calories, select a variety of foods from the major food groups (emphasizing those low in fat, salt, and sugars), and limit their intake of alcoholic beverages.

MEETING THE RECOMMENDATIONS

The general strategies described in this section for implementing dietary recommendations at the points of food purchase, preparation, and consumption are not meant to be comprehensive nor specific to any individual. Individuals' food choices differ on the basis of dietary preferences and dislikes, nutrient and energy needs, and many other factors (see Chapter 3). For example, an active college athlete with high caloric needs can eat more food than a sedentary roommate of the same sex and similar age and height who is restricting calories to reduce weight. If both roommates were to eat diets that meet the recommendations and contain the same percentage of calories from fat, carbohydrate, and protein, the higher-calorie diet of the athlete would contain a greater total amount of these macronutrients. In contrast, recommendations for cholesterol and sodium intake, which are given in absolute amounts, are the same for both. Because the athlete consumes more food than the dieter, the athlete will need to pay careful attention to limit intake of foods that are high in these nutrients.

The emphasis on consuming certain foods and limiting others is based on common dietary practices in the United States as shown by food consumption surveys. People who already consume diets that meet some or all of the *Diet and Health* recommendations should be encouraged to continue their healthful eating habits and make specific modifications as appropriate.

Implementors have important roles to play in helping people to apply the principles of dietary recommendations when they shop for food, prepare meals, and eat outside the home. In addition, implementors should encourage people to take political and other actions that will lead to health-promoting food choices becoming more widely available and being perceived as desirable choices (see Chapter 8).

Table 4-1 presents a general guide for meeting dietary recommendations. Consumers can use this guide along with other information in this chapter and a variety of publications from the U.S. Department of Agriculture (USDA) and the U.S. Department of Health and Human Services (DHHS) (see, for example, NCI/NHLBI, 1988, and USDA, 1989) to eat in ways that meet dietary recommendations as well as the RDAs.

Food Selection

Wise food shoppers select a variety of foods from all the major food groups, emphasizing those within each group that are low or relatively low in fat, salt, and simple sugars. By planning menus in

TABLE 4-1 Guide to Meet Dietary Recommendations[a]

Food Group	Recommended Number of Servings
Grains and legumes	At least six servings per day; consume grains in their whole form as often as possible. A serving is equivalent to one slice of bread or one small roll; 0.5 bun, bagel, or muffin; 0.5 cup of cooked cereal, rice, or pasta; 1 oz of ready-to-eat cereal; or 0.5 cup of cooked legumes.
Vegetables and fruits	At least five servings per day, with an emphasis on a variety of green and yellow vegetables (e.g., broccoli, kale, sweet potatoes, and carrots) and citrus fruits (e.g., oranges and grapefruits). A serving is equivalent to 0.5 cup of fresh or cooked vegetables or fruits, 1 medium fresh fruit or vegetable, 1 cup of leafy raw vegetables, 6 oz of juice, or 0.25 cup of dried fruit.
Dairy products	Two servings per day for children, three to four servings per day from ages 11 to 25 and for pregnant and lactating women, and two to three servings per day from age 25. A serving is equivalent to 8 oz (1 cup) of milk or yogurt, 1.5 oz of natural cheese, and 2 oz of processed cheese.
Meat, poultry, fish, and alternates (eggs, legumes, nuts, and seeds)	Two servings per day. A serving is equivalent to approximately 3 oz (cooked weight) (4 oz raw) of lean meat, fish, or poultry. Count 1 egg, 0.5 cup of cooked legumes, or 2 tablespoons of peanut butter as 1 oz of meat. Limit egg yolks to no more than three to four per week; there are no limits on egg whites.
Other foods (fats, sweets, and alcohol)	Limit use of foods that are high in oil, fat, or simple sugars; limit use of these items in food preparation. For those who drink alcoholic beverages, limit consumption to less than 1 oz of pure alcohol per day.

[a]This guide has been constructed from the following sources: DHHS, 1990; NRC, 1989a,b; and USDA, 1989. Modest differences exist among these sources in the way foods are grouped (e.g., in the placement of legumes) and in the recommended number of servings from each group (e.g., should there be a minimum recommended number of servings for both vegetables and fruits?). Nevertheless, they are very similar in the general type of eating pattern recommended.

advance and preparing a list of needed items before shopping for food, consumers may decrease impulse buying (particularly of foods with high levels of dietary components that should be limited) and stay within their food budgets. Shoppers should be encouraged to read nutrition labels to help them choose health-promoting products.

Food Preparation

The nutritional quality of foods can be affected by preparation methods. For example, the potential reduction in fat intake achieved by skinning a chicken breast may be more than offset if a high-fat sauce is served. The fat content of the latter could be greater than that in an equivalent amount of top round steak that is carefully trimmed and then broiled. As a general rule, frying of foods is discouraged; low- or no-fat alternatives include steaming, broiling, roasting, baking, boiling, stewing, microwaving, and stir-frying (if little oil is used).

Time-constrained cooks may find it easier to prepare quick yet nutritious meals with the help of appliances such as the microwave oven, pressure cooker, crockpot (slow cooker), blender, and food processor. Time can also be saved by purchasing presliced fruits, vegetables, and meats, which are increasingly available in supermarkets, but at extra cost. Cooks should be encouraged to use recipes that call for no or only small amounts of fatty, salty, or sugary items as essential ingredients or flavor enhancers.

Eating Outside the Home

People have limited control over the preparation of foods when they eat out, but they can select the types and the amounts of foods to be consumed. Full-service restaurants usually provide the largest selection of menu items prepared in a variety of ways compared with the expanding but still limited menus in fast-service food establishments.

People should be encouraged to choose restaurants that honor special requests and to inform the waitstaff how they want their meals to be prepared and served. Implementors should also provide consumers with tips for eating out, such as the following: if serving sizes of the entrees seem too large, ask for half or petite portions, choose an appetizer as a main dish, or share the entree; order fish, poultry, or meat broiled without fat, and poultry without skin; ask that salad dressings and sauces be served on the side; ask about the availability of foods that may not be on the menu such as skim milk or fresh fruit; and balance any high-fat or high-salt items with foods that are lower in these components.

The limited menus of fast-service food establishments—where an estimated 20% of the U.S. population eats on a typical day (Massachusetts Medical Society Committee on Nutrition, 1989)—make it difficult for people to select meals at these places that are low in fat and salt, since so many products are fried and seasoned. Consumers should be encouraged to order small sandwiches (such as single hamburgers rather than special, larger ones with special sauces), select prepared vegetable salads or items from the salad bar if available and use low-calorie dressings, and ask for low-fat or skim milk, fruit juice, or water as beverage options.

Many resources are available to help consumers put dietary recommendations into practice by improving their skills in selecting and preparing foods. They include cookbooks and books on diet and health; booklets and pamphlets issued by the federal government (particularly the Human Nutrition Information Service of the USDA), the Cooperative Extension Service (CES), voluntary health agencies, and several food retailers; community nutrition education classes sponsored by local high schools, colleges, and universities or by CES; and cooking classes. Professional nutritionists and dietitians are often knowledgeable about these resources and can be contacted by the public at local hospitals or health departments. These health-care professionals are trained to help individuals who need special assistance to improve or fine-tune their dietary patterns or to overcome personal difficulties in meeting dietary recommendations.

This committee recommends that additional resources be prepared. These include a comprehensive manual to assist consumers in incorporating the principles of dietary recommendations into their eating patterns and a food skills, nutrition, and health curriculum to teach children such concepts from an early age (see Chapter 8).

ACHIEVING SPECIFIC DIET AND HEALTH RECOMMENDATIONS

(1) Reduce total fat intake to 30% or less of calories. Reduce saturated fatty acid intake to less than 10% of calories and the intake of cholesterol to less than 300 mg daily.

According to the Committee on Diet and Health, a large and convincing body of evidence from studies on humans and laboratory animals shows that diets low in saturated fatty acids (saturated fat) and cholesterol are associated with low risks and rates of atherosclerotic cardiovascular diseases. High-fat diets are also linked to a high incidence of some types of cancers (especially of the colon, prostate, and breast) and probably obesity. That committee noted that there is

TABLE 4-2 Total Fat, Saturated Fat, and Cholesterol Intake in the Average U.S. Diet Compared to the *Diet and Health* Recommendations

Intake	Total Fat, % of total kcal	Saturated Fat, % of total kcal	Cholesterol, mg
Diet and Health recommendation for people from age 2 year[a,b]	≤30.0	<10.0	<300
Men (19 to 50 years old)[c]	36.4	13.2	435
Women (19 to 50 years old)[c]	36.7	13.4	272
Children (1 to 5 years old)[c]	34.9	14.0	233

[a] From NRC (1989a).

[b] The average nutrient intake by the U.S. population cannot be directly compared with the quantities specified in the *Diet and Health* recommendations, because the latter are goals for individuals. For example, if the goal for mean total fat intake by individuals is ≤30% of kcal, then the mean intake by the population would have to be substantially below 30% of kcal to achieve an intake of 30% by all people from age 2 (unless, of course, they all consumed exactly 30% of their calories from fat). Thus, the quantitative gap between this recommendation and the current intake by the U.S. population is wider than is apparent from the table.

[c] From USDA (1986c, 1988).

sufficient evidence that even further reductions in intake of total fat, saturated fat (to 8 or 7% of calories), and cholesterol (to 250 or 200 mg or even less per day) might confer even greater benefits. It concluded, however, that its recommended levels are more likely to be adopted by the public because they can be achieved without drastic changes in usual dietary patterns and without undue risk of nutrient deficiency (NRC, 1989a).

Table 4-2 presents the total fat, saturated fat, and cholesterol intake by adult men and women ages 19 to 50 and of children ages 1 to 5 as determined by recent USDA surveys (USDA, 1986c, 1988). It shows that total fat and saturated fat intake in the U.S. population will need to be reduced substantially if this most important of the *Diet and Health* recommendations is to be met. In addition, men will need to reduce their cholesterol intake, whereas the intake of many women and children appears to be within the recommendations. Since many people will find it difficult to make the dietary changes required to meet this recommendation overall, implementors face the challenge of educating and motivating them to action.

The major dietary sources of total fat, saturated fat, and cholesterol in the United States are meats (especially beef and pork); processed or convenience meat products (e.g., hot dogs and luncheon meats); whole-milk dairy products (e.g., milk, cheese, and ice cream); eggs; fats and oils (butter, margarine, mayonnaise, and salad and cooking oils); and grain-based but fat-rich products such as doughnuts, cookies, cakes, and crackers (Block et al., 1985). Altogether, animal products—which include red meats (beef, lamb, pork, and veal), poultry, fish and shellfish, separated animal fats (such as tallow and lard), milk and milk products, and eggs—contribute more than half of the total fat in U.S. diets, three-fourths of the saturated fat, and all the cholesterol (NRC, 1988).

Consumers will be better prepared to compare food products and evaluate promotional claims if they learn the difference between the percentage of fat by weight in a product and the percentage of calories from fat. Percentage of fat by weight refers to the quantity of fat in a product divided by the total weight of the product (which includes components such as carbohydrate, protein, and alcohol, if present, that supply calories to the diet as well as noncaloric water—an ingredient found in substantial amounts in most foods, even in solid or dry ones). In contrast, the percentage of calories from fat refers to the number of calories from a food supplied by fat divided by the total number of calories (from carbohydrate, protein, fat, and alcohol) supplied by the food. The value for percentage of fat by weight is lower—often substantially lower—than the value for percentage of calories from fat. The difference is based largely on the water content of the product. For example, ground beef labeled *extra lean* that contains 16% fat by weight would derive more than 53% of its calories from fat. Two percent milk contains 2% fat by weight (most of the rest of its weight is water), but 36% of its calories come from fat. It should be remembered, however, that as long as the total fat content of the diet remains within 30% of total calories, the percentage of calories from fat in any food product is not important. There is room for some high-fat foods in low-fat diets.

One practical strategy for reducing total fat, saturated fat, and cholesterol in the diet is to limit the consumption of meat, fish, and poultry to 3 oz cooked weight (about the size of a deck of playing cards) at any meal and to a maximum of approximately 6 oz/day. This action will also help to keep protein intake at recommended levels. USDA surveys show that total intake of meat, poultry, and fish averages 9.5 oz for adult men ages 19 to 50 (USDA, 1986c) and 5.4 oz for women of the same age range (USDA, 1988). Following are information and guidelines for selecting meat, poultry, and fish products to help meet this particular *Diet and Health* recommendation:

General
  • Meat, poultry, and fish provide essential nutrients. Meat is an especially good source of iron and zinc.
  • Poultry and fish are generally lower in fat compared with beef or pork.
  • USDA regulations allow fresh cuts of meat and poultry to be labeled *extra lean* if they contain no more than 5% fat by weight and *lean* or *low fat* if they contain less than 10% fat. Even most of the leanest meats, however, provide substantially more than 30% of their calories as fat. Fully trimmed lean beef, for example, supplies from 29% (for top round) to 41% (for tenderloin) of calories from fat after cooking (Beef Industry Council and Beef Board, 1990).
  • Choose the leanest looking cuts of meat and poultry and remove visible fat on the outside of the cut and between the muscles.

Meat
  • The leanest cuts of beef include round tip, top loin, top round, eye of round, tenderloin, and sirloin (Beef Industry Council and Beef Board, 1990).
  • The leanest cuts of pork include tenderloin, loin chops, and smoked ham (Giant Food, Inc., 1988).
  • Most trimmed cuts of veal, except the breast, are considered to be lean. The leanest cuts of lamb include the trimmed leg and loin (e.g., loin chops) (Giant Food, Inc., 1988).
  • When buying graded beef, choose the *select* grade (formerly known as *good*) over that labeled *choice* or, especially, *prime*. Select contains less intramuscular fat (known as marbling) than choice or prime beef.

Ground Beef and Turkey
  • Ground beef, the single largest source of fat in U.S. diets (Block et al., 1985), is exempt from USDA definitions of *lean* and *extra lean* meats. Even ground beef labeled *extra lean* is a relatively fatty product, which after cooking is approximately 16% fat by weight and derives more than 53% of its calories from fat (NRC, 1988). To minimize fat intake from ground beef, drain off the fat after cooking. In meatloafs and other dishes where the fat cannot be drained, use ground sirloin.
  • Ground turkey is lower in fat than ground beef (about 7 to 14% by weight) (Giant Food, Inc., 1988), but commercially available products get approximately 45% of their calories from fat because manufacturers grind up the turkey skin with the meat (Nutrition Action, 1989b).
  • To obtain a lower-fat alternative to prepackaged ground beef or turkey, select a lean cut of meat or skinned turkey breast and ask the butcher to grind it.

Organ Meats
  • These products derive at least one-quarter of their calories from fat and are particularly high in cholesterol. Each ounce of cooked beef liver, for example, derives 27% of its total calories from fat and supplies 110 mg of cholesterol (USDA, 1986a).

Poultry
  • Skinless turkey contains less fat than chicken. In roasted white meat, 7% of total calories is provided by fat compared with 23% in dark meat (USDA, 1979).
  • Removing the skin from chicken reduces the amount of calories from fat from 44 to 23% in cooked white meat and from 56 to 42% in dark meat (USDA, 1979).
  • Roasting a chicken breast without skin rather than frying it reduces the amount of calories from fat from 22 to 19% (USDA, 1979).

Luncheon or Deli Meats
  • Because these products are usually high in fat and sodium, their consumption should be limited. Sliced roast beef, turkey, or lean ham are relatively low-fat choices. Processed meats that are at least 95% fat free by weight are preferable; however, even a 95% fat-free ham with 23 calories per slice still contains 35% of calories as fat. Approximately 80% of the calories in beef hot dogs come from fat; turkey or chicken hot dogs are marginally lower (approximately 70%) (USDA, 1979, 1986a).

Fish and Seafood
  • The fat content of these foods is low to moderate and is largely unsaturated. In particular, fatty fish (such as salmon, mackerel, and tuna) supply n-3 fatty acids, which lower triglyceride levels when substituted for saturated fatty acids (NRC, 1989a). Consumption of fish one or more times per week has been associated with a reduced risk of coronary heart disease.
  • Compared with tuna canned in water or brine, tuna in oil contains up to 500% more fat and more than double the percentage of calories from fat (37 compared with 17%) (NRC, 1988).
  • Broiling rather than breading and frying a lean halibut steak reduces the amount of calories from fat from 47 to 18% (NRC, 1988).

Frozen Entrees
  • These popular products usually contain meat or poultry combined with a sauce, grain, vegetable, and sometimes a dessert. As a general rule, an entree containing less than 10 g of fat is likely to derive less than 30% of its calories from fat. According to a recent survey, the product lines of numerous frozen entree manufacturers ranged from 14 to 54% of total calories from fat; many are also high in sodium (Liebman, 1988a).

Dairy products are a major source of total fat, saturated fat, and cholesterol in the diets of the U.S. population. They are also the major food source of calcium, a nutrient in short supply in the diets of many adolescent and adult women. To limit fat and cholesterol intake from dairy products, one must switch from whole-milk products to those made with skim or low-fat milk. Following is a list of information and guidelines for use in selecting these foods:

Milk
- Canned evaporated skim milk or skim milk can be used in place of cream or whole milk.
- Substituting skim milk for whole milk (which derives almost 50% of its calories from fat) saves 8 g of fat per cup. Eight ounces of 2% milk (2% fat by weight but 36% fat as a percentage of total calories) and 1% milk (17% of calories from fat) contain 5 and 2 g of fat, respectively.

Cheese
- Because most natural hard cheeses (those made directly from milk) contain approximately 8 g of fat and 100 kcal/oz, more than 70% of their calories are derived from fat. Many supermarkets carry natural cheeses (such as cheddar, Colby, and Swiss) that contain about one-third less fat and fewer calories than their regular versions; typically, skim milk replaces some of the whole milk in these products (Liebman, 1989a; Nutrition Action, 1989a).
- Lower-fat versions of mozzarella, ricotta, cottage cheese, cream cheese, and sour cream are available.
- Processed cheeses are lower in fat than are natural hard cheeses, because some of the cheese is replaced with lower-fat ingredients. However, they are usually higher in sodium (Tufts University, 1988).

Yogurt
- Yogurts made with skim or low-fat milk are widely available.

Ice Cream
- Ice creams usually contain substantial amounts of fat and sugar. Premium ice creams contain from 400 to 450 kcal/0.75-cup serving and 24 to 27 g of fat. Regular ice creams containing less butterfat provide 220 to 235 kcal per serving and 11 to 13 g of fat. Substitutes include ice milk (170 to 190 kcal/0.75-cup serving; 5 to 7 g of fat), sherbet (205 kcal/serving; 3 g of fat), and sorbet (170 kcal/serving; virtually no fat) (Burros, 1989). Sherbet and sorbet, however, provide little or no calcium.
- Other alternatives to fat-rich ice creams include frozen yogurt (120 to 190 kcal/0.75-cup serving; 0 to 5 g of fat) and ice cream-like fat-free frozen desserts (50 to 70 kcal/serving; some of them supply calcium) (Liebman, 1989b).

Additional sources of dietary fat are fats and oils, nuts, some grain-based products, and snack foods. Information and guidelines for decreasing fat intake from these sources are provided in the following list:

Fats and Oils
- Butter, margarine, cooking and salad oils, and mayonnaise derive al-

most all their calories from fat; each teaspoon supplies 5 g of fat containing approximately 45 kcal. Limiting the use of these products can decrease the fat content of the diet substantially, as can the substitution of lower-fat versions of these products (e.g., imitation mayonnaise, vegetable oil spreads, diet margarine, and whipped butter).

• The use of nonstick cookware and vegetable oil sprays will reduce the need for fats and oils in cooking.

• Fat-reduced and fat-free salad dressings are available in supermarkets and sometimes in restaurants.

• Saturated fat intake can be lowered by substituting vegetable oils and margarine (whose major ingredient is liquid vegetable oil) in place of butter and lard.

Nuts

• An average of 84% of the caloric content of nuts (including peanuts) is provided by fat, but less than 20% of it is saturated. One exception is chestnuts; only 8% of their calories are contributed by fat. One ounce of pistachios (about 25 nuts), for example, contains 16 g of fat and 172 kcal (USDA, 1984).

Grain Products

• Some grain-based products are very high in fat, as a result of the fats added during preparation. Thus, consumption of croissants, doughnuts, cakes, and pies should be limited.

• Approximately 40% of the caloric content of an average cookie, and as much as 60% of some cookies, is provided by fat. Cookies that derive less than 30% of their calories from fat include graham crackers, ginger snaps, animal crackers, and fig newtons (Quint, 1987).

• Crackers vary in fat content; those that feel greasy to the touch are highest in fat. Low-fat crackers include rice cakes, crisp breads, matzo, melba toast, and zwieback.

• Granola cereals are particularly high in fat.

• Limit the intake of pasta and rice dishes prepared with cream, butter, or cheese sauces.

Snack Foods

• These products are often high in fat (although relatively low in saturated fat, since vegetable oils high in polyunsaturates are used in their preparation) and sodium. Potato chips and corn chips usually contain from 8 to 11 g of fat per ounce (50 to 60% fat calories), whereas tortilla chips obtain from 40 to 50% of their calories from fat (Schmidt, 1989). "Light" chips may be somewhat lower in fat.

• Among commercial snack foods, the lowest in fat is pretzels, since they are baked (Schmidt, 1989). The most fatty pretzels (3 g/oz) still contain half the fat of the least fatty potato chips.

• Popcorn can be a low-fat snack if it is air popped without the addition of oil (90 kcal/3 cups popped) or sprinkled with very small amounts of margarine or butter. In contrast, commercially available microwave popcorns contain considerably more fat per serving, averaging 56% of their calories from fat (Liebman, 1988b). Microwave popcorn products with fewer calories, fat, and salt have become available (Johnson and Erickson, 1989).

In the United States, the major source of dietary cholesterol by far is egg yolk, each of which contains approximately 215 mg of cholesterol. Cholesterol intake from egg-containing foods such as bakery products can be reduced by substituting one-and-a-half to two egg whites for each whole egg in most recipes. Acceptable egg entrees can usually be prepared by using one egg yolk with two or three egg whites. Also available are commercial egg substitutes consisting almost entirely of egg whites. Meat, poultry, and dairy products supply most of the remaining cholesterol in the U.S. diet. Consuming skim or low-fat dairy products in place of whole milk and products made from it will lower dietary cholesterol intake. Because organ meats tend to be very high in cholesterol, their use should be limited.

Some people may find it useful to establish a *fat budget* as a means to reduce their intake of total fat and saturated fat. A fat budget is established by determining one's caloric needs and deciding on a particular target for percentage of caloric intake from fat and saturated fat. For example, a 2,000-kcal diet that meets the *Diet and Health* recommendations could obtain 30% of its calories from fat and 9% of total calories from saturated fat. The total fat allowed with this diet would be limited to 67 g, no more than 20 g of which could come from saturated fat. Total fat and saturated fat intake could then be calculated by using the nutrition labels on food products, tables of food composition contained in basic nutrition textbooks and several government publications, and lay nutrition books that provide nutrient values of food. Professional nutritionists and registered dietitians can help interested individuals to establish fat budgets.

Alternatively, one can approximate total fat intake by using a system established for diabetics and overweight people to enable them to comply with their special diets. In this system, foods are placed into one of six *exchanges*; a serving of food within each exchange contains approximately the same amount of fat, carbohydrate, and protein (ADA and ADA, 1986, 1989). For example, one serving from the fat exchange (e.g., 1 teaspoon of butter, margarine, or mayonnaise or 1 tablespoon of salad dressing) contains approximately 5 g of fat and 45 kcal. Use of the exchange system to reduce fat intake will almost automatically lead to reductions in saturated fat and cholesterol intake as well. Booklets describing the exchange system are available from the American Dietetic Association in Chicago, Illinois, and the American Diabetes Association in Alexandria, Virginia.

With or without a fat budget, implementors should encourage

consumers to compare the fat content of food products within categories (e.g., milk and frozen meat entrees) and generally to choose those containing less fat as often as possible. For example, one 8-oz cup of whole milk contains 8 g of fat (more than 10% of the total of 67 g allowed in the example of a 2,000-kcal diet discussed above), but a cup of skim milk contains only a trace. Likewise, 1 oz of a high-fat meat like bratwurst contains 8 g of fat in contrast to the 3 g in 1 oz of lean meat such as select-grade flank steak or chicken.

(2) Every day eat five or more servings of a combination of vegetables and fruits, especially green and yellow vegetables and citrus fruits. Also, increase intake of starches and other complex carbohydrates by eating six or more daily servings of a combination of breads, cereals, and legumes.

The Committee on Diet and Health recommended that healthy adults and children from age 2 increase their carbohydrate intake to more than 55% of total calories by eating more carbohydrate-containing foods. These include grains, legumes (dried beans and peas), and vegetables (which contain starch or complex carbohydrates) as well as fruits (which contain natural sugars or simple carbohydrates). (Serving sizes of carbohydrate-rich foods are provided in Table 4-1.) These foods are generally low in fat, and therefore good substitutes for fatty foods, and are good sources of numerous vitamins, minerals, and dietary fiber. The Committee on Diet and Health recommended limiting the intake of products with added sugars (simple carbohydrates), which are strongly associated with dental caries and contain few nutrients. Furthermore, food products that contain large amounts of added sugars (e.g., pastries and ice cream) are often high in fat as well. Some, such as sherbet and many candies, contain little or no fat, but are very low in most essential nutrients.

The Committee on Diet and Health found that studies in various parts of the world indicate that people who habitually consume a diet high in plant foods have low risks of cardiovascular diseases, probably in large part because such diets are usually low in animal fat and cholesterol. Some constituents of plant foods, such as soluble fiber and vegetable protein, may also contribute—to a lesser extent— to the lower risk of cardiovascular diseases. That committee also noted that frequent consumption of vegetables and fruits, especially green and yellow vegetables and citrus fruits, is associated with decreased susceptibility to cancers of the lung, stomach, and large intestine. The mechanism is unknown, but it may be related to the carotenoid or dietary fiber content of these foods or to various other nutritive and nonnutritive components. In addition, produce is a good source of potassium; high intakes of this nutrient (approximately 3.5 g/day or more) may contribute to reduced risk of stroke, which is especially common among blacks and older people of all races.

Recent dietary surveys show that adult men in the United States consumed 45.3% of their calories as carbohydrates; the corresponding percentages for adult women and for children of both sexes from ages 1 to 5 were 46.4 and 52%, respectively (USDA, 1986c, 1988). Many people who eat at least the recommended number of servings of fruits, vegetables, grains, and legumes will automatically increase the total carbohydrate and complex carbohydrate content of their diets. Surveys show that many people do not consume enough fruits and vegetables. The second National Health and Nutrition Examination Survey (NHANES II), conducted from 1976 through 1980, indicated that on any given day the variety and amounts of fruits and vegetables consumed were limited: 49% of the nationally representative sample of adults ate no "garden vegetables" (all vegetables except potatoes, dried beans and peas, and salad), and only 20% ate a vegetable rich in vitamin A (such as green and yellow vegetables). Also, 41% of the sample ate no fruit, and only 28% consumed a vitamin C-rich fruit (such as citrus) or vegetable (Patterson and Block, 1988). In a survey conducted in California in 1989, 35% of adults reported eating two or fewer total servings of fruits and vegetables on the previous day; 7% ate no foods from this category (California Department of Health Services, 1990). Forty percent reported that only three or fewer servings of these foods should be eaten every day for good health.

Some vegetables and fruits should be consumed in their fresh, raw state; produce locally available in season is likely to be at the peak of its nutritional value and rich in flavor. Whole fruits and vegetables are generally preferable to juices, since the latter are not as rich in fiber and nutrients. Grains should be consumed in their whole form whenever possible. Whole-grain products such as whole-wheat bread, brown rice, and oatmeal retain the nutrient- and fiber-rich endosperm and bran of the plant; enriched or fortified grains do not contain all the nutrients or, usually, the fiber of the whole grain.

This committee also recommends that most people increase their consumption of legumes. Legumes—dried beans and peas such as black beans, pinto beans, kidney beans, navy beans, soybeans, black-eyed peas, split green or yellow peas, chick peas (garbanzos), and lentils—are good, inexpensive foods often described as meat alternates because they are rich in protein and other nutrients found in meat (e.g., B vitamins and trace elements). Most are rich in complex carbohydrates and dietary fiber and are low in fat. One cup of cooked kidney beans, for example, contains less than 1 g of fat (4% of total calories). Following is a compendium of information and guidelines on the selection and preparation of vegetables, fruits, grains, and legumes:

Vegetables

• Vegetables can be consumed either raw or cooked and can be purchased fresh, frozen, and canned.

• Green and yellow vegetables to emphasize in the diet include carrots, broccoli, winter squash, spinach, kale, and collard greens.

• For maximum nutrient retention, vegetables should be cooked in minimal amounts of water and only until they reach the tender but still crisp stage. Overcooking leads to excessive nutrient losses and loss of firm texture. They can be seasoned, if desired, with herbs, spices, lemon juice, or small amounts of margarine or butter.

• Minimize consumption of vegetables that are fried or served with sweet or fatty sauces.

• Minimize use of salad dressings on salads.

• Vegetables can be cooked with meats in roasts, stews, soups, and in various one-pot combination dishes.

Fruits

• Fruits, like vegetables, can be consumed either raw or cooked (such as baked or broiled) and can be purchased fresh, frozen, and canned. Fruits are also frequently consumed as juices.

• Citrus fruits to emphasize in the diet include oranges, tangerines, and grapefruit.

• Frozen and canned fruits packed in their natural juices or very light syrup are preferred to those packaged in sugar or heavy syrup.

Grain Products

• Grains can be combined with many other foods (e.g., meat, poultry, fish, and cheese), thus helping to reduce the fat content of the dish.

• Most breads and cereal products are low in fat; notable exceptions include croissants, pastries, cakes, and granola, which are prepared with fat.

• Rice or pasta can be combined with lightly sautéed vegetables, legumes, and perhaps with small amounts of meat along with herbs and spices to make nutritious low-fat entrees; the use of cream, butter, and cheese sauces on these entrees should be limited.

Legumes

• Legumes are versatile; they can frequently replace (or be added to) meat or poultry in combination dishes or be consumed alone or in salads.

• Cooked beans and peas are available in cans or frozen packages, fostering quick and convenient preparation. Draining and rinsing them before use will reduce substantially their content of sodium and simple sugars that come from the packaging liquid. Canned refried beans contain added fat; the type of fat (e.g., saturated fat-rich lard and coconut oil or the largely unsaturated safflower oil) varies by brand.

(3) Maintain protein intake at moderate levels.
The Committee on Diet and Health reported that there are no known benefits from and possibly some risks in consuming diets rich in animal protein. It noted that increased risks of certain cancers (especially those of the breast and colon) and heart disease have been associated in some population studies with diets high in meat (and, therefore, in animal protein) and with high protein intake alone in laboratory studies. That committee concluded, however, that it is not known whether these adverse effects are due solely to the usually high total fat, saturated fatty acid, and cholesterol content of diets that are rich in meat or animal protein or to what extent protein per se or other factors also contribute to these adverse effects. The Committee on Diet and Health recommended that total protein intake not exceed twice the RDA for all age groups. Table 4-3 can be used to determine this maximum recommended intake.

Approximately two-thirds of the protein in U.S. diets comes from animal products and one-third comes from plants. The main sources

TABLE 4-3 RDAs for Protein and Maximum Recommended Intakes[a]

Category	Age, years	RDA, g/kg	Median Weight, kg	RDA, g/day	Maximum Recommended Intake (2× RDA),g/day
Children, both sexes	2-3	1.2	13	16	32
	4-6	1.1	20	24	48
	7-10	1.0	28	28	56
Males	11-14	1.0	45	45	90
	15-18	0.9	66	59	118
	19-24	0.8	72	58	116
	≥25	0.8	79	63	126
Females	11-14	1.0	46	46	92
	15-18	0.8	44	44	88
	19-24	0.8	58	46	92
	≥25	0.8	63	50	100

[a] The RDA for protein ranges from 1.2 g/kg (2.2 lb) of body weight for children ages 2 to 3 to 0.8 g/kg for adults past age 18 (approximately 0.54 and 0.36 g of protein per pound of body weight, respectively). For those within the range of ideal body weight for height, the maximum recommended protein intake (twice the RDA) can be calculated by multiplying one's weight in kilograms by the appropriate RDA as g/kg and then multiplying that result by 2. Those who are substantially underweight or overweight can approximate their RDA for protein by using the median weights in column 4.

TABLE 4-4 Approximate Protein Content of Foods

Food Product	Serving Size	Amount of Protein, g/serving
Milk or yogurt	1 cup	8
Cheese	1 oz	8
Meat, poultry, and fish	1 oz	7
Whole egg	1	6
Legumes	0.5 cup cooked	5
Cereals and pasta	0.5 cup cooked	3
Bread	1 slice	3
Starchy vegetables	0.5 cup cooked	3
Vegetables	0.5 cup cooked or 1 cup raw	2

SOURCE: ADA and ADA (1986, 1989).

are fresh and processed meats, dairy products, and grains (particularly bread, rolls, and crackers) (Block et al., 1985). According to a recent survey, men from ages 19 to 50 consumed an average of 98 g/day, whereas women in the same age range and their children ages 1 to 5 averaged 61 and 53 g/day, respectively (USDA, 1986c, 1988). These average protein intakes are substantially greater than the RDAs but less than twice the RDA, suggesting that the majority of people in the United States already meet this dietary recommendation. Those who eat large amounts of meats and dairy products may, however, consume protein at levels higher than twice the RDA. Most foods, except fruits and purified fats and sugars, contribute some protein to the diet (see Table 4-4).

The Committee on Diet and Health recommended that protein intake not be increased to compensate for the calories lost in cutting back on fat in the diet. Protein intake can be maintained at moderate levels (between the RDA and twice the RDA) by limiting intake of meat, fish, and poultry to 6 oz or less per day while consuming at least six servings of grains and legumes and five servings of fruits and vegetables. Modest reductions in protein intake that may occur by modifying dietary patterns to meet dietary recommendations should be of no nutritional consequence to most healthy people.

(4) Balance food intake and physical activity to maintain appropriate body weight.

The Committee on Diet and Health reported that excess weight is associated with an increased risk of several disorders, including noninsulin-dependent diabetes mellitus, hypertension, coronary heart disease, osteoarthritis, and endometrial cancer. The risks appear to decline following a sustained reduction in weight. Increased abdominal fat carries a higher risk for these disorders than do comparable fat deposits in the hips and thighs.

That committee noted that body weight and body mass index are increasing in the U.S. population and other westernized societies, whereas caloric intake is decreasing. The undesirability of continuing this trend as well as the proven association of moderate, regular physical activity with reduced risks of heart disease led that committee to recommend that people in the United States increase their physical activity, improve physical fitness, and moderate their food intake to maintain appropriate body weight.

As part of a package of preventive health care, implementors of dietary recommendations should encourage and help people to engage in regular physical activity and to improve their eating habits. Exercise programs can be tailored to individuals with the help of qualified health-care professionals. All healthy people can work some exercise into their daily lives, from walking more often to taking the stairs up or down one or two flights rather than riding an elevator. Successful exercise programs are composed of activities that are convenient, enjoyed, and fit to one's routine schedule and physical abilities or limitations.

Because fat contains more than twice the calories of equal amounts of carbohydrates or protein, attempts at weight loss may succeed with a strategy that combines increased physical activity with a reduction in caloric intake by replacing foods high in fat with low-fat alternatives or other foods that are rich in complex carbohydrates but relatively low in fat. Moderate physical activity on a regular basis should be considered an essential component of any biologically rational and safe weight loss program. Regular activity helps to guard against excessive weight gain that tends to occur with aging and enables those at desirable weights to eat more food, thereby increasing the nutritional quality of the diet if food choices are made in accordance with the principles of dietary recommendations.

(5) The committee does not recommend alcohol consumption. For those who drink alcoholic beverages, the committee recommends limiting consumption to the equivalent of less than one ounce of pure alcohol in a single day. This is the equivalent of two cans of beer, two small glasses of wine, or two average cocktails. Pregnant women should avoid alcoholic beverages.

The Committee on Diet and Health reported that excessive alcohol consumption increases the risk of heart disease, hypertension, chronic liver disease, some forms of cancer (of the oral cavity, pharynx, esophagus, and larynx, especially in combination with cigarette smoking), neurological diseases, nutritional deficiencies, and many other disorders. Even moderate drinking carries some risks in circumstances that require neuromotor coordination and judgment, e.g., when driving vehicles and working around machinery. In addition, consumption of even small amounts of alcohol can lead to dependence. The Committee on Diet and Health noted that a causal association has not been established between moderate alcohol drinking and a lower risk of coronary heart disease. It specifically recommended against alcohol consumption by pregnant women because of the risk of damage to the fetus and the fact that no safe level of alcohol intake during pregnancy has been established.

There is approximately 0.40 oz of pure alcohol (ethanol) in a 12-oz bottle or can of most U.S. beer (which ranges from 3.2 to 4.0% ethanol by volume), a 3.5-oz glass of wine (from 11 to 13% ethanol in most table wines), and 1 oz of 80 proof (40% alcohol) distilled spirits such as whiskey (NRC, 1989a). These amounts should be considered one serving. To limit ethanol consumption to less than 1 oz/day, alcoholic beverage consumption should be limited to no more than two servings per day. Those who drink more potent alcoholic beverages—malt liquor beers containing more than 4% ethanol, fortified wines such as sherry and port that may contain approximately 20% ethanol, or distilled spirits greater than 80 proof—should limit themselves to less than two servings per day.

Alcoholic beverages such as wine or vermouth may be used in cooking to sauté or flavor foods. Until recently, it was believed that the ethanol was evaporated by the heat of cooking, but recent research shows that up to 85% of it may remain in the heated entree (Science News, 1989). Thus, pregnant women and others who wish to avoid ethanol should refrain from cooking with alcoholic beverages. As a practical matter, however, a negligible amount of ethanol is consumed from a dish cooked with up to several tablespoons of an alcoholic beverage and thus need not be considered.

(6) Limit total daily intake of salt (sodium chloride) to 6 g or less.

According to the Committee on Diet and Health, studies of human populations around the world have shown that diets containing more than 6 g of salt per day are associated with elevated blood pressure. While susceptibility to salt-induced hypertension is probably genetically determined, no reliable genetic marker has yet been identified. Therefore, the salt-sensitive individuals who are likely to benefit most from this recommendation cannot yet be identified. That committee concluded that this recommendation to limit salt intake would have no detrimental effect on the general population.

The Committee on Diet and Health recommended limiting salt intake to 6 g (6,000 mg) or less per day as a practical and achievable goal for people in the United States. It noted, however, that a greater reduction in salt intake (i.e., to 4.5 g or less) would probably confer even greater health benefits. Since salt is 40% sodium by weight, 6 g of salt is equivalent to 2.4 g (2,400 mg) of sodium. One teaspoon of salt (5 g) contains 2,000 mg of sodium.

Salt intakes by the U.S. population are difficult to determine, partly because of difficulties in measuring salt added during cooking and at the table. Data from a variety of sources suggest that total daily per capita intake in the United States ranges from 10 to 14.5 g. About one-third of this is estimated to be provided naturally in foods, one-third is added during food processing, and one-third is added at home during cooking or at the table (NRC, 1989a). A careful study in Great Britain, however, indicates that only 10% of dietary salt intake was naturally present in foods, whereas 15% came from salt added during cooking and at the table and fully 75% came from salt added during processing and manufacturing (Sanchez-Castillo et al., 1987a,b).

To meet this dietary recommendation, many people will need to make substantial changes in the foods they eat and in the ways they prepare them. Specifically, the consumption of processed foods that contain high levels of added sodium or are salt-preserved and salt-pickled should be limited. Most modern processing methods increase sodium and reduce the potassium content of foods. For example, the sodium content of 1/2 cup of fresh green peas is 2 mg; those same peas frozen or canned would contain approximately 70 and 186 mg of sodium per ounce, respectively (USDA, 1984).

White bread, rolls, and crackers supplied the most sodium in U.S. diets, according to NHANES II (Block et al., 1985), since sodium is added in manufacturing these products. Processed meats including hot dogs, ham, and luncheon meats were the second largest contributors of sodium. Given the high sodium content of many processed foods, more than 6 g of salt might be consumed, for example, simply by eating several frozen prepared pancakes for breakfast, a can of soup for lunch, and a frozen entree for dinner.

To reduce salt intake to recommended levels, consumers should study food product labels to identify product choices within categories (e.g., soup and cereals) that are lowest in sodium (and fat). Under current regulations, products may carry the term *sodium free* if they contain less than 5 mg of sodium per serving; products labeled *very low sodium* and *low sodium* must not exceed 35 and 140 mg per serving, respectively. Products labeled *reduced sodium* must contain at least 75% less sodium than the regular version of the product (IOM, 1990). For example, tomato puree labeled *no salt added, unsalted,* or *without added salt* contains approximately 50 mg of sodium per cup compared with 1,000 mg/cup in the version with added salt (USDA, 1984). Salt-containing canned vegetables, legumes, and other products can be drained and rinsed to remove some of their sodium. One study showed that rinsing canned green beans for 1 minute before heating them in water removed 40% of their sodium and that rinsing water-packed tuna for the same length of time decreased its sodium content by 76 to 79% (without simultaneously reducing the iron content) (Vermeulen et al., 1983).

Many consumers may not realize that products that do not taste salty may still contain considerable amounts of salt. For example, a single ounce of ready-to-eat breakfast cereal may contain more than 300 mg of sodium (Consumer Reports, 1989). A serving of apple pie at a fast-service food establishment may contain more than twice the sodium of a regular order of salted fries (Jacobson and Fritschner, 1986). Unless a food product lists its sodium content on the label, it will be difficult for most people to learn this information from other sources.

In addition to limiting the intake of many processed foods, salt intake can be reduced by minimizing its use at the table and in food preparation. Foods on the plate should always be tasted before salting, of course, but home cooks may not realize that salt can often be omitted or reduced in recipes without affecting their taste adversely. Lemon juice and salt-free seasonings consisting of herbs or spices alone or with dried vegetables are recommended alternatives to salt. Some consumers may find the use of *light* salts to be a helpful interim measure; they contain potassium chloride in addition to sodium chloride and supply approximately half the sodium of regular salt.

High sodium intakes are most commonly associated with diets high in prepared, processed foods or with heavy discretionary use of table salt. Low intakes of sodium are associated with diets consisting largely of fresh fruits, vegetables, cooked legumes, and grain products— foods that naturally contain little sodium. Dairy products contain moderate levels of sodium. An 8-oz glass of milk supplies about 120 mg (USDA, 1976); most natural cheeses contain between 100 and 400 mg/1.5-oz serving (Liebman, 1986). Generally, natural hard cheeses are lower in sodium than processed cheeses, cheese foods, and cheese spreads. Unprocessed cereal grains such as oats and brown rice are very low in sodium, although products made from them (e.g., ready-to-eat cereals) may contain substantially more (pasta is a notable exception). For example, one slice of enriched white bread or whole-wheat bread contains from approximately 65 to 160 mg of sodium per slice (Consumer Reports, 1988). Rich baked goods are often high in sodium as well as in fat and simple sugars. Generally, fresh meats, poultry, and fish supply less than 90 mg of sodium per 3-oz serving, while the same size serving of processed meat such as sausages, luncheon meat, and frankfurters contain from 750 to 1,350 mg (USDA, 1986d).

Since the dietary recommendation to limit salt intake is independent of caloric intake, the ease of compliance is likely to depend on the amount of food consumed; it is easier to limit sodium intake when consuming 1,500 compared with 3,500 kcal/day. Those with high caloric needs may not be able to meet this recommendation unless special measures are undertaken to curtail the use of processed foods and the salt shaker.

(7) Maintain adequate calcium intake.

The Committee on Diet and Health recommended that food choices be made to obtain adequate calcium, a nutrient essential for proper growth, development, and maintenance of the bones. Certain segments of the U.S. population are susceptible to inadequate calcium intake, especially adult women because of their low caloric intake and adolescents because of their high requirements for this mineral. RDAs for calcium are 800 mg/day for children through age 10 and for adults beyond age 24. RDAs increase to 1,200 mg/day for adolescents from ages 11 through 24, the critical years of bone mass accretion, and for pregnant and lactating women, to meet the calcium needs of their offspring.

Dairy products are rich sources of calcium. They contribute more than 55% of the calcium intake of the U.S. population (Block et al., 1985). Skim, low-fat, and whole milk contain equivalent amounts of calcium, approximately 300 mg/cup (USDA, 1976). Thus, calcium intake can be maintained while total fat and saturated fat are being reduced by dietary patterns that include the use of skim and low-fat milk. Most hard cheeses contain from 100 to 200 mg of calcium per ounce (Dairy Nutrition Council, Inc., 1989). People who cannot or do not drink milk should be encouraged to eat cheese or yogurt (which contains approximately 300 mg of calcium per cup). Lower-fat versions of these products and yogurt made with nonfat milk are available.

Calcium intakes in the United States are low for groups other than adult men. The most recent national survey indicated that the average daily calcium intakes of adult men and women ages 19 to 50 and of children ages 1 to 5 were 919, 621, and 824 mg, respectively (USDA, 1986c, 1988). Nutrition educators frequently recommend that older children, adolescents, and young adults consume 3 cups of milk per day or its equivalent in other dairy products to supply approximately 75% of the RDA for calcium from this group, and it is recommended that adults from age 24 consume the equivalent of 2 cups/day. Non-fat dry milk powder, which contains 377 mg of calcium in 0.25 cup (USDA, 1976), can be added to recipes (e.g., small amounts to baked goods and meatloafs) to provide additional calcium.

Nondairy sources of calcium include green vegetables, such as collards (218 mg/1 cup chopped, raw), kale (90 mg), mustard greens (58 mg), and broccoli (42 mg) (USDA, 1984). Other calcium-containing foods include tofu prepared with calcium, lime-processed tortillas, the soft bones of fish such as salmon and sardines, and calcium-fortified foods (NRC, 1989b). One orange contributes 52 mg of calcium (USDA, 1982); cooked legumes can provide 35 to 80 mg/cup (USDA, 1986b).

(8) Avoid taking dietary supplements in excess of the RDAs in any one day.

As noted by the Committee on Diet and Health, vitamin and mineral supplements are taken by a large percentage of the U.S. population every day; they are often self-prescribed and their use is not usually based on known nutrient deficiencies. The committee recognized that some population subgroups (e.g., those suffering from malabsorption syndromes) may require supplements and recommended that they be used only under professional supervision.

Most healthy people who eat diets that are in conformance with dietary recommendations and that contain adequate calories will come close to meeting or exceed the RDAs for nutrients and therefore have no need for supplements. As stated earlier, RDAs are defined as levels of intake of essential nutrients judged to be adequate to meet the known nutrient needs of practically all healthy people. Because RDAs include a margin of safety, they exceed the actual requirements of most people. Therefore, people who do not consume RDA levels of all nutrients are not likely to be malnourished. Those concerned about the nutritional quality of their diet should consult a qualified health-care professional for an evaluation; if a supplement is indicated, one can be recommended that will compensate for nutrients in short supply in the diet.

Consumers who choose independently to take dietary supplements should limit themselves to products that do not contain excessive amounts of any nutrients. Label information pertaining to the U.S. Recommended Daily Allowances (USRDAs) can be used to evaluate and compare products. USRDAs are a set of values developed by the Food and Drug Administration on the basis of the 1968 (seventh) edition of the RDAs (NRC, 1968) to be used as standards for the nutritional labeling of foods and dietary supplements. The USRDAs are generally the highest RDA values for each nutrient (excluding values for pregnant and lactating women) given in that edition, in which nutrient allowances were generally higher than they are in the most recent (tenth) edition (NRC, 1989b). Thus, USRDAs are very generous standards. A healthy person who takes a daily supplement containing 100% of the USRDA for nutrients will probably consume—from food and the supplement—some vitamins and minerals at levels two to three times his or her RDAs and thus will very likely exceed his or her actual nutrient requirements. These levels, while not known to be harmful, are unlikely to confer better health.

(9) *Maintain an optimal intake of fluoride, particularly during the years of primary and secondary tooth formation and growth.*
The Committee on Diet and Health recommended that people of all ages consume water with a natural or added fluoride content ranging from 0.7 to 1.2 parts per million to reduce the risk of dental caries. Drinking such water is especially important for children during the years of primary and secondary tooth formation and growth. In the absence of optimally fluoridated water, that committee supported the use of dietary fluoride supplements in amounts recommended by the American Dental Association, the American Academy of Pediatrics, and the American Academy of Pediatric Dentistry (these levels are summarized in NRC, 1989a).

REFERENCES

ADA and ADA. (American Dietetic Association and the American Diabetes Association, Inc.). 1986. Exchange Lists for Meal Planning. American Diabetes Association, Alexandria, Va. 32 pp.

ADA and ADA. (American Dietetic Association and the American Diabetes Association, Inc.). 1989. Exchange Lists for Weight Management. American Dietetic Association, Chicago, Ill. 33 pp.

Beef Industry Council and Beef Board. 1990. Advertisement: What's the skinny on beef? Cooking Light 4:16s.

Block, G., C.M. Dresser, A.M. Hartman, and M.D. Carroll. 1985. Nutrient sources in the American diet: quantitative data from the NHANES II survey. II. Macronutrients and fats. Am. J. Epidemiol. 122:27-40.

Burros, M. July 5, 1989. Ancient, ever-fresh sorbets. New York Times. C1, C4.

California Department of Health Services. 1990. 1989 California Dietary Practices Survey, Focus on Fruits & Vegetables. Highlights. Nutrition and Cancer Prevention Program, California Department of Health Services, California Public Health Foundation. Nutrition and Cancer Prevention Program, Sacramento, Calif. 37 pp.

Consumer Reports. 1988. Your daily bread. Consumer Reports 53:611-614.

Consumer Reports. 1989. Cereal: breakfast food or nutritional supplement? Consumer Reports 54:638-646.

Dairy Nutrition Council, Inc. 1989. A Cheese Lover's Guide to Low Fat Cheeses. Dairy Nutrition Council, Inc., Westmont, Ill. 6 pp.

DHHS (U.S. Department of Health and Human Services). 1990. Healthy People 2000: National Health Promotion and Disease Prevention Objectives. Conference edition. Public Health Service, U.S. Department of Health and Human Services. U.S. Government Printing Office, Washington, D.C. 672 pp.

Giant Food, Inc. 1988. Eat for Health: Meat Guide. Form 233 (3/89 CMX). Giant Food, Inc., Landover, Md.

IOM (Institute of Medicine). 1990. Nutrition Labeling: Issues and Directions for the 1990s. Report of the Committee on the Nutrition Components of Food Labeling, Food and Nutrition Board. National Academy Press, Washington, D.C. 355 pp.

Jacobson, M.F., and S. Fritschner. 1986. The Fast-Food Guide. Workman Publishing, New York. 225 pp.

Johnson, B., and J.L. Erickson. 1989. Popcorn leaders make light moves. Advertising Age 60(32):2.

Liebman, B. 1986. "Low-fat" cheeses. Nutr. Action Healthletter 13(2):10-11.

Liebman, B. 1988a. Frozen finds: a survey of light meals. Nutr. Action Healthletter 15(1):10-11.

Liebman, B. 1988b. Popcorn primer. Nutr. Action Healthletter 15(7):10-11.

Liebman, B. 1989a. Dairy lightens up. Nutr. Action Healthletter 16(2):10-11.

Liebman, B. 1989b. Frozen fantasies. Nutr. Action Healthletter 16(5):10-11.

Massachusetts Medical Society Committee on Nutrition. 1989. Fast-food fare: consumer guidelines. N. Engl. J. Med. 321:752-756.

NCI/NHLBI (National Cancer Institute/National Heart, Lung, and Blood Institute). 1988. Eating for Life. NIH Publication No. 88-3000. U.S. Government Printing Office, Washington, D.C. 23 pp.

NRC (National Research Council). 1968. Recommended Dietary Allowances, 7th edition. Report of the Food and Nutrition Board, National Research Council. Publication 1694. National Academy of Sciences, Washington, D.C. 101 pp.

NRC (National Research Council). 1988. Designing Foods: Animal Product Options in the Marketplace. Report of the Committee on Technological Options to Improve the Nutritional Attributes of Animal Products, Board on Agriculture. National Academy Press, Washington, D.C. 367 pp.

NRC (National Research Council). 1989a. Diet and Health: Implications for Reducing Chronic Disease Risk. Report of the Committee on Diet and Health, Food and Nutrition Board, Commission on Life Sciences. National Academy Press, Washington, D.C. 749 pp.

NRC (National Research Council). 1989b. Recommended Dietary Allowances, 10th Edition. Report of the Subcommittee on the Tenth Edition of the RDAs, Food and Nutrition Board, Commission on Life Sciences. National Academy Press, Washington, D.C. 284 pp.

Nutrition Action. 1989a. Cheese for a lifetime. Nutr. Action Healthletter 16(8):16.

Nutrition Action. 1989b. Ground turkey vs. ground beef. Nutr. Action Healthletter 16(2):13.

Patterson, B.H., and G. Block. 1988. Food choices and the cancer guidelines. Am. J. Public Health 78:282-286.

Quint, L. 1987. A cookie compendium. Nutr. Action Healthletter 14(10):10-11.

Sanchez-Castillo, C.P., S. Warrender, T.P. Whitehead, and W.P. James. 1987a. An assessment of the sources of dietary salt in a British population. Clin. Sci. 72:95-102.

Sanchez-Castillo, C.P., W.J. Branch, and W.P. James. 1987b. A test of the validity of the lithium-marker technique for monitoring dietary sources of salt in men. Clin. Sci. 72:87-94.

Schmidt, S.B. 1989. Salty snacks. Nutr. Action Healthletter 16(4):10-11.

Science News. 1989. More than a taste of alcohol. Science News 136:318.

Tufts University. 1988. Say 'cheese,' but with discretion. Tufts Univ. Diet & Nutr. Letter 6(10):7.

USDA (U.S. Department of Agriculture). 1976. Composition of Foods. Dairy and Egg Products: Raw, Processed, Prepared. Agriculture Handbook Number 8-1. Agricultural Research Service, U.S. Department of Agriculture. U.S. Government Printing Office, Washington, D.C. 144 pp.

USDA (U.S. Department of Agriculture). 1979. Composition of Foods. Poultry Products: Raw, Processed, Prepared. Agriculture Handbook No. 8-5. Science and Education Administration, U.S. Department of Agriculture. U.S. Government Printing Office, Washington, D.C. 330 pp.

USDA (U.S. Department of Agriculture). 1982. Composition of Foods. Fruits and Fruit Juices: Raw, Processed, Prepared. Agriculture Handbook No. 8-9. Human Nutrition Information Service, U.S. Department of Agriculture. U.S. Government Printing Office, Washington, D.C. 283 pp.

USDA (U.S. Department of Agriculture). 1984. Composition of Foods. Vegetables and Vegetable Products: Raw, Processed, Prepared. Agriculture Handbook No. 8-11. Nutrition Monitoring Division, U.S. Department of Agriculture. U.S. Government Printing Office, Washington, D.C. 502 pp.

USDA (U.S. Department of Agriculture). 1986a. Composition of Foods. Beef Products: Raw, Processed, Prepared. Agriculture Handbook No. 8-13. Nutrition Monitoring Division, Human Nutrition Information Service, Hyattsville, Md. 396 pp.

USDA (U.S. Department of Agriculture). 1986b. Composition of Foods. Legumes and Legume Products: Raw, Processed, Prepared. Agriculture Handbook No. 8-16. Nutrition Monitoring Division, Human Nutrition Information Service, Hyattsville, Md. 156 pp.

USDA (U.S. Department of Agriculture). 1986c. Nationwide Food Consumption Survey. Continuing Survey of Food Intakes of Individuals. Men 19-50 Years, 1 Day, 1985. Report No. 85-3. Nutrition Monitoring Division, Human Nutrition Information Service, Hyattsville, Md. 94 pp.

USDA (U.S. Department of Agriculture). 1986d. Nutrition and Your Health, Dietary Guidelines for Americans: Avoid Too Much Sodium. Home and Garden Bulletin No. 232-6. Human Nutrition Information Service, Hyattsville, Md. 8 pp.

USDA (U.S. Department of Agriculture). 1988. Nationwide Food Consumption Survey. Continuing Survey of Food Intakes of Individuals. Women 19-50 Years and Their Children 1-5 Years, 4 Days, 1986. Report No. 86-3. Nutrition Monitoring Division, Human Nutrition Information Service, Hyattsville, Md. 182 pp.

USDA (U.S. Department of Agriculture). 1989. Dietary Guidelines and Your Diet. Home and Garden Bulletin Nos. 232-8 through 232-11. Human Nutrition Information Service, U.S. Department of Agriculture, Hyattsville, Md.

Vermeulen, R.T., F.A. Sedor, and S.Y.S. Kimm. 1983. Effect of water rinsing on sodium content of selected foods. J. Am. Diet. Assoc. 82:394-396.

5

Public Sector: Strategies and Actions for Implementation

W HO SHOULD implement the growing consensus on dietary recommendations? Governments exist to provide for the common good and the welfare of their citizens—and by extension the public's nutritional health. Therefore, governments at all levels have special obligations to implement dietary recommendations both by example and by the unique actions that they can take.

Governments at all levels can promote implementation directly through legislation and rule-making; provision of information and education; awarding of research and demonstration grants; intramural research, education, and extension programs; food assistance and farm programs; their own vast meal service functions; and through acting as role models by providing examples of implementation in government facilities, by government officials, and at government-funded events. The public sector can also encourage this effort indirectly by setting an agenda for the implementation of various strategies, initiating dialogue with the private sector and voluntary organizations, and coordinating implementation efforts. This array of efforts must be pursued in the legislative and executive branches at federal, state, and local levels.

The committee focuses here on the role of the federal government, but it should be emphasized that many of the committee's recommendations are applicable at state and local levels as well. Moreover, it will be necessary for those who are intimately aware of the special characteristics of each local situation to apply them. Involvement by

112

state and local governments as well as other societal sectors discussed in this report is essential if implementation is to become a reality.

GOVERNMENTS AS IMPLEMENTORS

Throughout this chapter, reference is made to government activities under way to encourage people to eat healthful diets. These activities include provision of qualitative advice as found in *Dietary Guidelines for Americans* (USDA/DHHS, 1980, 1985, 1990) (hereinafter referred to as the *Dietary Guidelines* report) and quantitative recommendations from the National Cholesterol Education Program (NCEP, 1990) and in the report *Healthy People 2000: National Health Promotion and Disease Prevention Objectives* (DHHS, 1990a). The U.S. Department of Agriculture (USDA) issued suggestions to state school food service directors on ways to implement the *Dietary Guidelines* in their school lunch programs (see, for example, USDA, 1983). In addition, studies on human nutrition related to the *Dietary Guidelines* report have been undertaken by USDA (1987) and the National Institutes of Health (NIH) (NIH, 1989).

But there are formidable barriers to implementing dietary recommendations in the public sector, including politics, bureaucracy, and costs. The political obstacles to change include pressures from food producers, processors, distributors, retailers, and industry, and other interest groups who believe they would be adversely affected economically if dietary patterns were to change or if current food service functions were required to offer options that they believe would be less acceptable to consumers, although more desirable from the standpoint of dietary recommendations. Government farm subsidies can exacerbate the situation by encouraging the production of less desirable food alternatives. Cost is a major factor when nutritionally desirable foods are more expensive than alternative products.

None of these barriers is easily overcome. First, the outside pressures and the bureaucratic and economic barriers to change must be acknowledged by governments at all levels. Second, current practices and activities that could be modified to foster implementation need to be identified, modified appropriately, and the benefits of such change evaluated. Plans for achieving each of these steps should be developed in cooperation with all those who are influenced by, or have a special interest in, the outcomes. Development of these goals and plans will require patience, political skills, and good will on the part of public officials and others involved in the political process. One example of such a successful effort was the preparation of the report *Healthy People 2000: National Health Promotion and Disease Pre-*

vention Objectives (DHHS, 1990a). These national objectives were formulated through a public process that involved federal, state, and local governments as well as private and voluntary groups. The objectives were also published in draft form for public comment (DHHS, 1989). Such open and inclusive processes are needed in developing nutrition policy to ensure support by all sectors.

PRINCIPLES THAT SERVE AS A BASIS FOR IMPLEMENTATION

It is desirable that initiatives to implement dietary recommendations in the public sector adhere to a set of principles. These principles, described below, were developed by the committee to help public institutions make nutritionally desirable food choices available, identifiable, and acceptable. These principles have also been applied in devising many of the committee's other recommendations described in Chapters 6 through 8.

Provide Information and Education

Governments must initiate and participate in comprehensive programs to inform consumers about dietary recommendations and about ways to integrate them into eating patterns. For example, government cafeterias should provide information that identifies eating patterns that conform to dietary recommendations. In addition, consumers should be given advice on how to follow the principles of the recommendations wherever they eat; and food producers, processors, distributors, and retailers should be advised on how to make the recommendations apply at, for example, farms, processing plants, supermarkets, and eating facilities. Private- and voluntary-sector participation in similar activities is essential.

Ensure Freedom of Choice

Coercion in food choices is rarely acceptable, especially for people who are institutionalized in government facilities or who are otherwise dependent on the government for their basic economic support. Thus, although information on dietary recommendations and menus conforming to their principles should be offered, selection should be as much as possible the responsibility of each individual. When government agencies formulate eating patterns and develop menus to implement dietary recommendations in food assistance and other programs, every attempt must be made to ensure that the cost of the recommended diet does not appreciably exceed the alternatives.

Foster Long-Term Commitment and Incremental Approaches

Experience with clinical dietetics, clinical trials, and community-based intervention studies has shown that incremental change is the most successful way to achieve long-term dietary adherence (see Chapter 3). Thus, to fully implement dietary recommendations without major disruptions to the food system or people's current eating preferences, incremental changes will need to be encouraged over years or decades— not weeks or months. Food producers, processors, marketers, and caterers should be strongly encouraged to initiate incremental changes conforming to the principles of dietary recommendations over a 5- to 10-year schedule. More rapid change is, of course, desirable and should be attempted when feasible.

Facilitate Access to Health-Promoting Foods

The special obligation of governments to implement dietary recommendations extends beyond education and the provision and coordination of information. It also involves ensuring that every U.S. citizen has access to the foods that can be used to meet these recommendations. In all government food-service operations and in dining areas in all government-supported institutions, foods should be offered that can be used to meet dietary recommendations, thereby providing an example for the private sector. Consumers should be given menu choices, but among those choices there should be at least one that is identified as helping people to meet dietary recommendations. When alternatives cannot be made available, the set menu should be one that helps people meet dietary recommendations.

Present Healthful Eating in a Context of Total Health Promotion

Dietary changes are adjuncts to, not substitutes for, a comprehensive system of health promotion, disease prevention, disease treatment, nutrition support, and social welfare measures, including economic and food assistance. Because governmental institutions have a special obligation to provide access to the basic needs of daily life and health, they should present good eating patterns as one of many life-style factors, such as cessation of smoking, reducing blood pressure, achieving ideal body weight, lowering serum cholesterol, and increasing physical activity, that can decrease chronic disease risk.

Involve All Interested Parties

Public officials at all levels of governments should work with representatives of interest groups in the public, private, and voluntary sectors to implement dietary recommendations. Collaborative efforts are likely to be most successful when many different people support the change and believe that their efforts will turn out favorably for them.

Ensure Palatability of Healthful Diets

Food plans designed to meet dietary recommendations must be made appealing to consumers in order to be accepted. The committee recognizes that the population's taste preferences may gradually shift with increasing exposure to meals that help it to meet dietary recommendations, but menu revisions must consider people's present food preferences. In addition, the palatability and acceptability of menus based on the principles of dietary recommendations should be tested in target populations for prolonged periods (i.e., weeks or months, not days). Health-promoting meals must be at least as appealing as the meals they are replacing.

Encourage Convenience

Health-promoting meals should be relatively convenient in comparison with current offerings with regard to purchasing, preparation, delivery, and consumption. Any proposed menus (especially *least-cost* menus and food plans) based on the principles of dietary recommendations should be tested in populations to ensure that they are acceptably convenient and appealing before being disseminated. Planning, preparing, and perhaps serving new menus may be less convenient at first, but will become more routine over time.

Encourage the Incorporation of Health-Promoting Foods in Food Programs

Foods rather than vitamin and mineral supplements should serve as the sole sources of nutrients to meet dietary recommendations in government food programs. It would not be acceptable to this committee were the government to suggest as a cost-cutting measure the use of dietary supplements or their equivalent (highly fortified products) instead of the planning of menus which meet, or come close to meeting, the Recommended Dietary Allowances (RDAs) (see Chapter 4).

Implement the Recommendations with Minimal Disruption of Food Preferences

In implementing dietary recommendations, menus and meal plans that entail the fewest disruptions to current food preferences are preferable. In addition, choices within food groups should be preserved whenever possible. Occasionally, however, consumers may need to make major changes in food preferences. The key to success in these cases is mapping out gradual changes and providing the needed transition period.

STRATEGIES AND ACTIONS FOR THE PUBLIC SECTOR

The committee developed five strategies and associated actions to assist governments at all levels in promoting the nutritional health and welfare of the public.

STRATEGY 1: Improve federal efforts to implement dietary recommendations.

The full potential benefits of implementing dietary recommendations can be approached by a federally coordinated effort, collaboration with state and local governments, and participation of the private sector, professional and voluntary organizations, and consumer advocacy and community groups. The committee recognizes that the federal government has done much to encourage Americans to eat well; many of these activities are mentioned in this report. For example, it has prepared and distributed many reports and consumer information materials on diet and health (see, for example, NCI/NHLBI, 1988, and USDA, 1981, 1984, 1986b,c, 1988a, 1989a). In addition, governmentwide interagency committees were formed to coordinate activities related to nutrition monitoring and human nutrition research. Within USDA and the U.S. Department of Health and Human Services (DHHS), subcommittees serve as departmental focal points for coordinating the preparation and dissemination of information and publications and for providing technical assistance on dietary guidance. To date, however, there is no governmentwide nutrition policy that provides a coherent blueprint for fostering healthful dietary patterns.

ACTION 1: *The executive branch should establish a coordinating mechanism that would promote the implementation of dietary recommendations.*
The executive branch has taken steps to coordinate many of its nutrition-related activities by establishing specific inter-and intra-agency groups. The Interagency Committee on Human Nutrition Research,

which coordinates government-sponsored nutrition research, is co-chaired by an assistant secretary from both USDA and DHHS; it includes representatives from USDA, DHHS, Department of Commerce, Department of Defense, Agency for International Development (AID), National Aeronautics and Space Administration, National Science Foundation, Office of Science and Technology Policy, and the Department of Veterans Affairs (DVA). The Interagency Committee on Nutrition Monitoring, which works to enhance the effectiveness and productivity of federal nutrition monitoring efforts, is also cochaired by an assistant secretary from both USDA and DHHS. It consists of representatives of USDA, DHHS, AID, DOD, DVA, Bureau of the Census, and the Department of Labor.

Because most nutrition-related activities of the federal government take place in USDA and DHHS, both departments have established administrative structures to ensure that food and nutrition information emanating from their various agencies are consistent with the *Dietary Guidelines* report (U.S. Congress, House, 1989b). The Dietary Guidance Working Group at USDA, established in 1986, is composed of representatives of at least eight USDA agencies (e.g., the Cooperative Extension Service, the Human Nutrition Information Service, and the National Agricultural Library) (USDA, 1986a). Similarly, the Nutrition Policy Board Subcommittee on Dietary Guidance in DHHS, established in 1987, consists of representatives from the NIH, the Food and Drug Administration (FDA), and the Centers for Disease Control (CDC) (DHHS, 1990b; U.S. Congress, House, 1989b). Each group has a liaison representative from the other agency to promote consistent and complementary messages on dietary guidance.

In two important respects, however, the federal government's efforts to implement dietary recommendations are insufficient. First, the charters of the interagency coordinating committees restrict them to narrow areas. The four administrative structures described above are not empowered to assume responsibility for implementing dietary recommendations, an effort that involves much more than providing information on diet and health, conducting nutrition research, and monitoring the nutritional status of the food supply and U.S. population. Secondly, these four groups are frequently criticized for failing to fulfill their narrowly-defined missions. For example, there is still no comprehensive nutrition surveillance system in place to adequately monitor trends in dietary intake, determine the nutritional status and knowledge of the population (particularly among high-risk minority groups and the disadvantaged and homeless), and report results in a timely fashion (Nestle, 1990). Government publications on diet and health too often are not available in ample quantities at the community level or may be too expensive for many people to purchase. In addition, little priority may be given to the dissemination of these materials by the local agencies that sponsor implementation activities.

The lack of a coordinating mechanism at the federal level to implement dietary recommendations has had unfortunate consequences. In some cases, nutrition policy decisions are made in a fragmented manner that can result in policies that are inconsistent from a public health perspective. Federal policies on alcohol, farm subsidies for some commodities, and means of grading and payment for certain commodities (e.g., by fat content) are examples.

The heads of the agencies with responsibilities in food and nutrition need to establish a suitable mechanism to ensure that all their policies and programs directly or indirectly related to these areas are compatible with the principles of dietary recommendations. The mechanism will need to (1) coordinate government efforts to implement dietary recommendations, (2) maximize each agency's independent ability to promote these recommendations, (3) establish consistent food and nutrition policies across government agencies, and (4) initiate and encourage collaborative efforts between government and outside agencies (including the states, the private sector, and voluntary groups).

The committee suggests that the executive branch consider establishing a single, high-level entity to coordinate and direct government nutrition activities. This was proposed as early as 1969 at the White House Conference on Food, Nutrition, and Health (White House, 1970). As an example, a committee could be established for this purpose, composed of a very senior-level person from each of the eight relevant cabinet-level departments (Agriculture, Commerce, Defense, Education, Health and Human Services, Interior, State, and Veterans Affairs). The representatives would have a small professional and support staff and major responsibilities in their departments for some aspect of the food system or for feeding people.

ACTION 2: *Encourage members of the U.S. Congress and state legislative bodies to play active roles in the implementation of dietary recommendations.*

Legislative bodies have special opportunities and responsibilities to devote some of their attention, interest, insights, and expertise on matters that affect the diet and health of their constituents. Many members of the U.S. Congress are becoming more cognizant of the key role that dietary patterns play in the general well-being of the public. Bills introduced in Congress pertaining to food and nutrition cover a broad range of activities and include legislation to reauthorize food assistance programs and legislation related to food labeling, nutrition monitoring, nutrition research, commodity food distribution programs, health promotion and disease prevention programs, and education and training programs.

Members of the U.S. Congress can assist in efforts to implement dietary recommendations in the various agencies through oversight hearings, authorizations and appropriations, conference report language, and other legislative actions. Support from the legislative branch will encourage high-level administrators in the executive branch departments to give priority and resources to dietary recommendations in policy guidelines, technical assistance programs, education and information initiatives, and other activities addressing the food, nutrition, and health needs of consumers.

The farm bill, which comes before Congress every 4 to 5 years, should be reviewed and revised with dietary recommendations in mind. Nutrition educators, registered dietitians, physicians, and other health-care professionals, working through their associations, should advise Congress during these periodic reviews. The 1990 farm bill is a landmark piece of legislation that mandates policies and programs governing many areas relevant to dietary recommendations: (1) extending and revising agricultural price support and related programs (e.g., for milk and sugar); (2) providing for agricultural export, resource conservation, farm credit, agricultural research, and related programs (e.g., human nutrition research, extension service, and land-grant institutions); (3) continuing certain food assistance programs to low-income people (e.g., food stamps and commodity distribution programs); and (4) ensuring consumers an abundance of food at reasonable prices (e.g., through commodity promotion, research, and information) (U.S. Congress, House, 1990; U.S. Congress, Senate, 1990).

State legislatures have many opportunities to promote the implementation of dietary recommendations. In September 1989, for example, California enacted legislation (Assembly Bill No. 2109) mandating its State Department of Education to "develop and maintain nutrition guidelines for school lunches and breakfasts, and for all food and beverages sold on public school campuses" (California Legislature, 1989, p. 3). These "guidelines shall include guidelines for fat, saturated fat, and cholesterol, and shall specify that where comparable food products of equal nutritional value are available the food product lower in fat, or saturated fat, or cholesterol shall be used" (p. 3).

STRATEGY 2: Alter federal programs that directly influence what Americans eat so as to encourage rather than impede the implementation of dietary recommendations. This effort should affect food assistance, food safety, and nutrition programs, as well as farm subsidy, tariff, and trade programs.

The primary federal food assistance programs are administered by USDA and DHHS together with state governments and local agencies. Two nutrition services for older Americans (congregate meals and home-delivered meals) are administered at the federal level by DHHS; others (e.g., the Food Stamp Program, School Lunch and Breakfast programs, the Child Care Food and Summer Food Service programs, and the Special Supplemental Food Program for Women, Infants, and Children [WIC]) fall under the jurisdiction of USDA. State departments of education usually have responsibility for food programs serving children in schools, child-care centers, and summer recreation centers. State departments of health, welfare, and agriculture usually have responsibility for programs providing food stamps or supplemental foods to families or individuals. The meals programs for elderly people are administered by state and area agencies on aging.

The potential for reaching vast numbers of the country's citizens who receive benefits through these programs is tremendous. For example, the School Lunch Program serves lunch to 24 million children each day, about half of them from low-income families (U.S. Congress, House, 1989a). At present, the nutritional standard for meals served under this program is limited to the requirement that they meet one-quarter to one-third of the RDAs (NRC, 1989b) over time through the choice of foods within a prescribed meal pattern.

The committee recommends that nutrition guidelines for this and all other food assistance programs be tied to dietary recommendations in a practical fashion. Participants in these programs should be able, if they desire, to eat diets that meet dietary recommendations in the normal course of their day-to-day living and not only by extraordinary effort. They should be able to receive appealing and easy-to-understand educational materials (of appropriate levels of comprehension and cultural sensitivity) about dietary recommendations and how to improve their eating habits with the help of the foods supplied by various assistance programs.

ACTION 1: *Revise current USDA regulations governing the child and family nutrition programs to comply with dietary recommendations and train federal, regional, state, and local personnel administering the programs to implement the recommendations.*

Many implementation efforts can be achieved without legislative or regulatory changes, while others require changes in laws and regulations. The committee's recommendation to ensure that nutrition programs adhere to dietary recommendations is one that requires statutory and regulatory change. For example, while only the School Lunch Program must offer students whole milk *and* at least one of the following: low-fat milk, skim milk, or buttermilk, the other child nutrition programs (e.g., the Special Milk, School Breakfast, Summer Food Service, and Child Care Food programs) require only that milk be fluid and pasteurized and that it meet state and local standards. It may be unflavored or flavored whole milk, low-fat milk, skim milk, or cultured buttermilk. The committee supports requirements that options be made available, with the caveat that low-fat and skim milk not be served to infants and children under age 2 without direction by a pediatrician (see Chapter 4).

To ensure that government nutrition programs adhere to dietary recommendations, it will also be necessary to provide training and other forms of technical assistance to those who administer the programs. Designers of training programs must recognize that the United States has a very decentralized, heterogeneous, multiethnic, multicultural system, which makes implementation difficult. Managers and cooks in all child and family food assistance programs should be trained in all critical aspects of food preparation and services. At a minimum, they should be taught menu planning, food purchasing, food preparation, and service techniques that support dietary recommendations. Governments must encourage private-sector contributions to such training programs.

The WIC food packages for women and children from age 2 and older should be reviewed for conformance with the principles of dietary recommendations. Fruits, vegetables, whole-grain products, and legumes should be included whenever possible. The committee recognizes that uniformity and cost issues must be addressed in modifying the WIC package. Relevant government agencies working with WIC nutritionists should prepare information and educational materials for WIC recipients on healthful ways of feeding their families to meet dietary recommendations. These materials should include caveats concerning the applicability of these recommendations to infants and children under age 2 and should address special issues (e.g., alcohol consumption) related to the health of pregnant and lactating women.

Food Stamp Program allotments are based on the cost of the Thrifty Food Plan, a nutritionally adequate set of food allowances developed by USDA for people of very limited financial means (Cleveland and Kerr, 1988). However, the committee believes that many low-income families lack the money (owing to other high fixed costs like shelter and transportation); food planning, purchasing, and preparation skills; and knowledge of food and nutrition to follow the Thrifty Food Plan so as to ensure the consumption of nutritionally adequate diets that meet dietary recommendations. The committee believes that dietary change in healthful directions would probably be fostered among low-income families if food stamp allotments were to be based on a more generous standard, such as USDA's Low-Cost Food Plan. This plan is approximately 20% greater in cost than the Thrifty Food Plan and would enable the purchase of a greater variety of foods. Recently, the American Dietetic Association recommended that food stamp allotments be based on USDA's Moderate-Cost Food Plan (Hinton et al., 1990), which is 40% more costly than the Thrifty Food Plan.

ACTION 2: *Revise current regulations governing the Nutrition Program for Older Americans (which provides congregate meals and home-delivered meals) to conform to the principles of dietary recommendations and train federal, regional, state, and local personnel administering the programs accordingly.*
Aging is accompanied by a variety of changes that can compromise nutritional status (DHHS, 1988a,b). These changes may be physiologic (e.g., decrease in sense of smell and dental problems), psychologic (e.g., depression), economic (e.g., declines in income), and social (e.g., living alone or in an institution). Elderly people who consume diets that meet dietary recommendations will reduce their risks of developing many degenerative chronic diseases, especially if they have eaten well in the past and engage in other health-promoting behaviors.

General principles for training cooks and other food service personnel described in other sections of this report also apply here. In addition, menu plans for the nutrition programs that feed elderly people should (1) be ethnically and biologically appropriate for the low-energy intakes characteristic of this group; (2) be appropriate for, and adaptable to, the physical and biological limitations of elderly people in preparing their food; and (3) be compatible with dietary and drug therapies (e.g., should not lead to adverse drug-nutrient interactions, which are common among the elderly). The fact that most elderly people have limited incomes and live in small families also should be taken into account.

The nutritionist's position at the Administration on Aging's (AOA) central office in DHHS has remained unfilled for nearly a decade. This position was and is vital for implementing standards and providing technical assistance to nutrition programs for elderly people. The committee believes that this important position must be restored and the office fully staffed. The AOA needs a nutrition adviser at the federal level to assist its program operations with implementation of dietary recommendations.

The nutrition-related recommendations resulting from the Surgeon General's Workshop on Aging (DHHS, 1988b) as well as some of the specific nutrition-related programs at DHHS on healthy aging need to be implemented. Coordination between offices in USDA and DHHS (e.g., NIH, AOA, and CDC) and private-sector coalitions will be needed to accomplish this. The major goal is to emphasize healthful eating in the context of overall health promotion, disease prevention, and disease treatment.

The committee urges those segments of the private sector involved in providing food for food assistance and other government programs to take an offensive rather than a defensive stand in implementing dietary recommendations. Producers and distributors must more actively consider these recommendations in developing new and modified foods for the elderly and for those who are part of other food assistance programs.

ACTION 3: *USDA and DHHS should ensure that food and health programs serving all special populations conform to dietary recommendations.*

Several food assistance programs serve many special populations, including Native Americans and those of Puerto Rico and other U.S. territories. As an example, the two largest programs serving Indians are the Food Stamp Program (FSP) and the Food Distribution Program on Indian Reservations (FDPIR). As an alternative to food stamps, FDPIR provides commodity foods to eligible households located on reservations. Because of high unemployment rates and low incomes, the federal programs are the major source of food in many of these households. Reservations are often located in remote areas of the country where lands are not suitable for farming. As a result, many tribes cannot provide all their own food, especially when economic resources are limited.

From 1988 through 1990, the GAO investigated the effectiveness of public and private programs in alleviating hunger and promoting the nutritional welfare of residents on Indian reservations. In their two reports to Congress on this matter (GAO, 1989, 1990), GAO stated that four major diet-related health conditions existed on the reservations studied: obesity, diabetes, heart disease, and hypertension. It also noted that "Although USDA improved the nutritional content of the FDPIR food package in 1986, tribal and . . . Indian Health Service . . . officials believe that the fat and sodium content of many of the available food items should be reduced further" (GAO, 1989, p. 4). Furthermore, it stated, "Food assistance programs can improve diets on Indian reservations by making available more nutritious foods and nutrition education" (p. 6).

The important role of nutrition education to ensure that FDPIR and FSP recipients get help with their dietary needs also was mentioned in the GAO reports. The committee urges the federal government to keep this in mind when establishing priorities and time frames for upgrading the nutritional quality of commodities to meet dietary recommendations. The importance of the cultural relevance and compatibility with the concept of gradual change cannot be overemphasized in the implementation of this action. The committee also supports the provision of greater resources to the Indian Health Services in its work to decrease morbidity in the Native American population.

ACTION 4: *Ensure that the education and information components of the foregoing federal food assistance and nutrition programs are consistent with dietary recommendations.*

Each of the previously mentioned food assistance and nutrition programs does or should have a nutrition education component. The committee recommends that higher priority be given to implementing dietary recommendations in education programs throughout the United States. Suggestions for improving nutrition education are found in Chapters 7 and 8.

The USDA's Nutrition Education and Training (NET) Program, if adequately funded (see Chapter 8), could provide ample opportunity to accomplish this action for schoolchildren. Each fiscal year, the state education agencies must submit a plan for their NET programs for approval by the USDA. They base their plans on an ongoing assessment and evaluation of the plans from previous years. Some of the activities that should be built into the NET Program plan of each state include reaching all children in the state with information on diet and health, providing in-service training for school food-service management personnel, offering teacher training in nutrition, and disseminating information to school officials and parents. Some states, such as Texas, have evaluated the effectiveness of their NET Program (Roberts-Gray, 1987). The committee encourages such action, especially after dietary recommendations have been integrated into state plans and programs.

A spring 1989 survey among a nationally representative, randomly selected sample of district school food-service directors revealed a great deal of uncertainty concerning the scientific consensus on daily fat intake levels. Respondents reported having limited access to written materials or training programs explaining how to purchase (e.g., preparing specifications for supplies) or modify recipes to reduce fat content. They also frequently mentioned the need for improved education and training to help lower the fat content of school meals (Shotland, 1989).

Another important government education program is the Expanded

Food and Nutrition Education Program (EFNEP) of USDA's Cooperative Extension Service, which was started in 1968 to help low-income families in all states, especially those with young children, acquire the knowledge, skills, attitudes, and behavior changes necessary to improve their diets (Chipman and Kendall, 1989). In 1970, the program was extended to serve low-income youths in the 4-H Program. These youths are taught nutrition-related skills, enabling them to improve the adequacy of their diets. EFNEP home economists provide on-the-job training and supervise paraprofessionals and volunteers who teach the low-income homemakers and youths. The paraprofessionals often live in the communities where they work and enroll homemakers in individual or group teaching sessions (USDA, 1984).

Ethnically appropriate materials (e.g., food and nutrition information tailored to cultural subgroups) should be made more available to guide food selection in accord with the principles of dietary recommendations. The committee recognizes that money and other resources must be provided and that creative ways need to be devised to make these materials available to consumers.

Outreach efforts for many public assistance programs can assist in the dissemination of information on diet and health to low-income families in every county of the nation. Full funding on a continuing basis plus a high-priority status conferred at the departmental level is needed if these programs are to fulfill their mandate and keep the country's citizenry informed of new knowledge about diet and health.

ACTION 5: *Incorporate dietary recommendations into current rules and regulations governing commodity purchases.*

To stabilize the prices that farmers and ranchers receive for many of the foods they produce, the federal government purchases the surplus production and distributes such commodities at no or low cost to several food assistance programs. About 30% of the value of all foods purchased for school meals comes from surplus food commodities donated to schools by USDA or purchased by them at reduced prices (USDA, 1989b). Because many food-service directors rely heavily on government commodities to help them stretch their food budgets, the nutritional quality of school meals can depend greatly on the types of commodities received. In addition, numerous emergency food programs across the United States depend on government surplus food commodities provided through the Temporary Emergency Food Assistance Program.

USDA has already taken a number of steps to make commodity foods more compatible with the principles of dietary recommendations. Efforts have been made to lower fat content, restrict the use of highly saturated fat, provide whole grains and fresh fruit, and to purchase lower-fat foods and commodities with reduced levels of salt and sugar (USDA, 1989b). Despite these efforts, a national survey by the advocacy group Public Voice for Food and Health Policy revealed that school food-service directors view commodity foods as a real barrier to implementing dietary recommendations (Shotland, 1989). Two-thirds of the directors identified USDA's Commodity Donation Programs as major obstacles to reducing fat in menus. Subsequently, Public Voice evaluated school lunch programs in schools across the country to assess the availability of low-fat options (Morris, 1990). It concluded that "too much fat is being offered our children in school lunches" (p. 2) and made recommendations for improvement. The Citizens Commission on School Nutrition (1990) recently issued a report with recommendations for improving the nutritional quality of the school lunch program.

The committee recommends that USDA continue its efforts to bring the nation's donated and surplus foods programs into closer compliance with the principles of dietary recommendations whenever possible. For example, the programs might try to include more whole-grain products, fruits and vegetables, low-fat rather than high-fat cheeses, lean rather than high-fat meat, poultry, legumes, and low-sodium products. Health-care professionals in communities could advise local food-service directors about foods to purchase that would nutritionally complement the commodities received, enabling the preparation of menus that help people to meet dietary recommendations.

Dietary recommendations should be a consideration in specifying and awarding processing contracts between the agencies distributing or receiving donated and surplus foods and processors, who convert the donated foods into finished items such as pastas and bread. Contracts should specify the nutritional profile of the end product and the amount and proportion of its ingredients. The committee believes that dietary recommendations should serve as an important specification in these contracts.

STRATEGY 3: Change laws, regulations, and agency practices that have an appreciable but indirect impact on consumer dietary choices so that they make more foods to support nutritionally desirable diets available. Examples are food grading and labeling laws and standards of identity for a number of food products.

ACTION 1: *Improve food labeling and food description, production, and processing regulations to permit consumers to make better informed choices.*

Consumers cannot make informed food choices unless they know how their dietary patterns contribute to health and risk of disease and how to improve their diets. Without this knowledge, consumers cannot know whether they are meeting dietary recommendations or what kinds of dietary trade-offs they may need to make so they can keep eating some favorite high-fat foods. Nutrition information provided on food labels is perhaps the most important and direct means of conveying such information.

The current framework for the nutrition labeling of foods in the United States was established in 1973. Under current regulations, nutrition labeling is voluntary for manufacturers, unless a nutrient is added or a nutritional claim is made for a product. Regulation of food labeling is currently shared by two federal agencies: USDA for meat, poultry, and egg products and the FDA for all other foods. The Federal Trade Commission is responsible for food advertising (IOM, 1990). Among current concerns about food labeling are the proliferation of health claims, the lack of full nutrition labeling for macronutrients, the limited extent to which foods are covered by labeling, and its complexity for many consumers (see Chapter 8).

There is general consensus that food labels should be updated and modified to provide consumers with important information to assist them in choosing healthful diets. FDA and USDA have devoted considerable effort to studying the issues, drafting proposed modifications for the content and format of labels, and planning for reform. On July 19, 1990, for example, FDA proposed standard serving sizes for foods according to product category (Benton and Sullivan, 1990), an action the committee applauds. Congress has also shown considerable interest in food labeling by holding hearings, drafting legislation, and publicly calling for label improvements; it culminated in the passage of the Nutrition Labeling and Education Act of 1990, which was signed into law by the President in November 1990. The private sector and health-care professionals have also contributed importantly to the debate and process of reform. A recent report of the Food and Nutrition Board (IOM, 1990) provides a detailed overview of the U.S. system of food labeling and many recommendations to improve it. This committee urges implementation of the recommendations in that report as well as continued study of ways in which food labels can be used to improve dietary patterns.

ACTION 2: *Develop and adopt regulations governing food descriptions, grading, and nomenclatural practices.*

These regulations would relate to standards of identity and quality grades for products such as meat and milk. Appropriate federal agencies should support the following three specific components of this action item:

A. *Review standards of identity, changing or discontinuing them as appropriate. These standards should be consistent with and promote the principles of dietary recommendations.*

With the intent to prevent economic fraud, the Federal Food, Drug, and Cosmetic (FD&C) Act requires FDA to establish standards of identity that define the composition of certain foods. Under current provisions of the FD&C Act, it is very difficult to change a standard once it has been adopted (IOM, 1990). Therefore, some standards have not kept up to date with advances in food technology and nutrition. For example, fat was considered to be a valuable component of food at the time that most standards were adopted, so standards of identity for cheese are based largely on its fat content. A cheese product with lower fat than required by the standard must be named something other than cheese (although it need not be labeled "imitation" if it is not nutritionally inferior to the standardized food). Consumers may be less willing to try products that do not have standardized names, even though some of them may fit more easily into diets meeting dietary recommendations. FDA has sought comments on possible approaches to addressing problems with current food standards and will address this area under its current food labeling initiatives (Food Chemical News, 1990).

B. *Review price supports for milk and examine the implications of increasing the dollar value of the nonfat portion and reducing the dollar value of the butterfat portion while keeping milk price constant.*

Dairy products are a major food item in the U.S. diet, and there has been a gradual increase in the purchase of low-fat milk. If the population is to lower its fat intake to 30% or less of total caloric intake, more low-fat dairy products need to be made available. At present, however, the price for milk paid to producers is based on the butterfat content. As an initial step toward decreasing the butterfat content of milk, the committee recommends that USDA study the economic implications to consumers and the dairy industry of increasing the dollar value of the milk solids component and decreasing the dollar value of the fat component. Adjustments in the milk pricing system should provide an impetus to dairy producers to start breeding, feeding, and managing their herds for decreased fat production (NDC, 1989).

C. *Review and, if necessary, change quality grades of meat and develop uniform nomenclature for ground beef to make these products more compatible with dietary recommendations.*

The grading system for beef and lamb has rewarded fatty meat with appealing grade names that encourages producers to fatten animals and deters them from producing lean meat. The grades are a vestige of the time when well-marbled meat meant better meat to consumers. The grading system needs to be reviewed in light of modern knowledge of diet and disease relationships. In 1987, a positive change in the U.S. grading system was the renaming of U.S. Good grade to U.S. Select (Clarke and Wise, 1988). By establishing a more positive grade name, the meat industry was given an opportunity to improve marketing of beef with less marbling than that in the Prime or Choice grade. A similar beneficial change is the action by the USDA's Agricultural Marketing Service to alter the Institutional Meat Purchase Specifications (IMPS) for fresh beef (USDA, 1988b). IMPS are voluntary guidelines for cut definitions and trimming practices used by the meat industry to help standardize quality control procedures. The IMPS now call for more fat to be trimmed from various cuts of beef than was designated in the past. The external fat on cuts of beef such as steak was reduced from one-half to one-quarter inch, and for the first time, the term *practically free of fat* was quantified as meaning that at least 75% of lean meat is exposed on the surface of the cut.

A national standard for grading and labeling lean ground beef should be adopted. Currently, individual states and supermarkets set their own standard for *lean, very lean,* and other terms to describe ground beef, and the actual fat content can vary considerably. This confuses consumers who are trying to decrease the fat in their diets. National uniform standards for the fat content in ground beef should be developed.

ACTION 3: *Improve the nutritional attributes of animal products.*

In 1988, a committee of the National Research Council's Board on Agriculture released its report *Designing Foods* (NRC, 1988). Many of the policy and research recommendations to improve the nutritional attributes of animal foods are supportive of dietary recommendations (see Chapter 6). This committee therefore suggests that governments review the report and adopt those recommendations that have a direct impact on the implementation of dietary recommendations.

STRATEGY 4: Enable government feeding facilities to serve as models to private food services and help people meet dietary recommendations.

In their roles as major food-service providers, governments (especially the federal government) have responsibilities to set a good example by offering meals that help people to meet dietary recommendations. In addition to developing implementation and demonstration projects, governments can exercise their leadership and educational roles by serving as models for the voluntary, private, and public sectors. Such projects can be instructive to key institutions in the country, including corporations, colleges and universities, correctional facilities, and hospitals. Through the efforts of the secretary of DHHS, several federal government facilities might serve as model programs. The NIH Clinical Center, a "showcase" hospital, could make changes in all nontherapeutic diets. The cafeteria in Building 31 on the NIH campus in Bethesda, Maryland, serves the visiting biomedical community and hospital and would be an excellent locus for a model program that implements dietary recommendations. It is unrealistic to expect others to change when government agencies (and private institutions that depend largely on federal funding) do not do so themselves. The cafeteria in the Hubert H. Humphrey Building in downtown Washington, D.C., which serves high-ranking federal and other health-care personnel, and the cafeterias of USDA have recently implemented changes that are in accord with dietary recommendations and might serve as models to other government-managed eating places.

Several issues associated with the implementation of dietary recommendations require further study. It is crucial to have information on technical problems that might be experienced in demonstration projects (e.g., in private-, voluntary-, and public-sector settings) in order to develop more effective implementation strategies.

In the committee's judgment, two barriers confront the implementation of Strategy 4. Perhaps the most fundamental barrier is the lack of political will. In the case of smoking, governments acknowledged the scientific evidence linking the habit to heart disease, lung cancer, and other diseases and took actions to restrict or eliminate smoking in their facilities. The committee hopes that as governments become more convinced of the connections between diet and health, they will become more active in implementing the principles of dietary recommendations in their own feeding facilities. The second barrier to implementation is the possibility that the civil liberties of the less fortunate are being infringed, e.g., by limiting the choice of foods available to those who are dependent on governments for subsistence, such as patients in hospitals, the very poor, and prisoners. Ways of protecting the rights of these people while encouraging them to adopt healthful dietary practices must be found. One way to avoid even the appearance of taking advantage of the less fortunate is to start implementation programs among independent groups rather than the indigent and dependent. For example, employee dining rooms in government facilities should be tackled before attempts to implement dietary recommendations are made with the hospitalized or the poor.

ACTION 1: *The Office of the Secretary of the U.S. Department of Veterans Affairs (DVA) should direct its health-care personnel to follow dietary recommendations in all of its food and health care systems.*
During fiscal year 1988, the U.S. Department of Veterans Affairs (formerly the Veterans Administration) maintained a total of 172 medical centers (hospitals), 119 nursing homes, and 26 domiciles for veterans and treated more than 1 million patients in these facilities (DVA, 1989). The DVA should incorporate dietary recommendations into all aspects of their food operations —menu planning, food purchasing, preparation, and service. The present clinical nutrition and dietetic personnel should be retained in the DVA system to provide the technical assistance needed to implement dietary recommendations.

Federal agencies, such as NIH through its National Cancer Institute or National Institute on Aging, should collaborate with the DVA medical system to develop grant mechanisms to establish demonstration projects for implementing dietary recommendations and other activities directed toward achieving the national health promotion and disease prevention objectives of DHHS by the year 2000 (DHHS, 1990a). Likewise, DVA and private hospitals should work cooperatively as often as possible to develop and coordinate research and training initiatives to accomplish this particular action. More recommendations about the training of health-care professionals are discussed in Chapter 7.

Several specific steps can be taken to further strengthen the use of diet and health principles in the DVA system. The first priority should be implementation of dietary recommendations in the food environment for the well patients and visitors in the DVA system; sufficient choice of foods should be available so that those who want to eat in a manner consonant with dietary recommendations are able to do so. Changes in the diets of sick patients need to be made on a case-by-case basis, since other therapeutic considerations may take precedence. In addition, the following actions should be considered:

• Provide more central direction and support for clinical nutrition within the DVA system. Take more action to implement dietary recommendations in canteens within the DVA. Baseline surveys should be conducted to assess current implementation efforts in canteens and elsewhere in the DVA.

• Develop policies and guidelines for implementing dietary recommendations. Implementation plans must then be put into effect at local levels. Without the support of medical and nursing staffs, little is likely to be accomplished. The dietetic services have no direct responsibility over the cafeterias and canteens in the DVA system.

- Encourage grant proposals for research and demonstration grants that enhance implementation of dietary recommendations.

ACTION 2: *The surgeons general of the Army, Navy, and Air Force within the Department of Defense (DOD) should develop a plan for implementing dietary recommendations in all aspects of the DOD food and health-care systems.* The DOD feeds thousands of people each day. It offers meals in dining halls, in other eating facilities, and in the hospitals and clinics it operates around the world. Because of these huge feeding operations, DOD purchases immense quantities of food and thus has a large influence on the country's food supply. The DOD assistant secretaries for health and the surgeon general of each service are charged with maintaining the health and fitness of enlisted personnel and their families. Thus, DOD has many opportunities to provide good examples of implementing dietary recommendations. The committee commends the DOD for making substantial advances in addressing nutritional concerns of military personnel over the past two decades. Since 1985, there has been an evaluation of the systems of feeding military populations to determine the nutritional adequacy of the diets consumed (DHHS, 1989). Results of this assessment serve as the basis for modifying menus, standardizing recipes, designing cook training programs, and developing specifications for the purchase of food and combat rations. In a recent assessment of basic Army trainees at Fort Jackson, South Carolina, mean dietary fat intakes by both the men and women for 7 days were less than 35% of total calories. The "absence of a short-order line and limitation on high-fat, high-calorie bakery items (donuts, pastries, etc.) may have assisted in the attainment of this goal" (U.S. Army, 1989). This assessment represents a single evaluation in a highly controlled environment. More attention needs to be paid to continuing evaluation, surveillance, and implementation of all aspects of dietary recommendations rather than on fat consumption alone.

Nutrition-related regulations for the nation's active and reserve military services have been in existence for decades. These regulations have three major purposes: (1) to establish dietary allowances for military feeding, (2) to prescribe nutrient standards for packaged rations, and (3) to provide basic guidelines for nutrition education. They were last revised in 1985 and will be reviewed again now that the 3rd edition of the federal government's *Dietary Guidelines for Americans* report (USDA/DHHS, 1990) has been released. Because these regulations are used by cooks in the military as well as by the vendors who supply packaged rations, the committee recommends that the manual of regulations provide more emphasis on practical ways to meet dietary recommendations. Special efforts must be made to motivate cooks and vendors to alter their products and make them more compatible with the principles of dietary recommendations.

ACTION 3: *The DOD's food and beverage services and practices should be revised to conform to dietary recommendations.*
Mess halls, officers' clubs, clubs for enlisted personnel, and other private food services on military facilities should be encouraged to serve at least one identified meal choice, among the several offered, that conforms to the principles of dietary recommendations. The committee believes that the DOD should also develop a plan to implement dietary recommendations in its food and health services, including canteens and officers' clubs. The emphasis should not be placed upon changing combat rations or other special feeding situations. The enormous complexity of the implementation process within the DOD is recognized. Yet at the very least, efforts in DOD facilities should match those of other federal facilities.

ACTION 4: *Urge the director of the Federal Bureau of Prisons to examine the feasibility of providing diets in line with dietary recommendations, recognizing the complexity of the correctional system and the special role of food in correctional facilities.*
The Federal Bureau of Prisons is responsible for ensuring the adequacy and healthfulness of diets served in the large network of federal correctional facilities under its jurisdiction. The social milieu of correctional institutions is complex, and changes in prison life are difficult to administer. Food has a great deal of symbolism in correctional institutions, and the mess hall is a place where violence occurs. Occasionally, correctional officials have instituted diets limiting sugary and sweet foods in the hope that they will prevent or treat violent and disruptive behavior, but this has been to no avail (Gray, 1986). The American Correctional Association, which reviews correctional facilities, suggests that menus meet the RDAs. These menus should also help prisoners to meet dietary recommendations. Groups including registered dietitians, nutrition educators, health educators, correctional officials, and inmates should convene to discuss and take action on designing acceptable prison diets that meet dietary recommendations.

ACTION 5: *The General Services Administration (GSA) should ensure that food contracts and monitoring systems are made to conform to the principles of dietary recommendations.*
Those who work in or visit government offices often dine in federal facilities. Others attend catered functions sponsored by govern-

ment agencies. Many government cafeterias are operated by the GSA, which in turn contracts with providers of food, catering, and vending services. Technical assistance to food producers and preparers should be provided or built into GSA contracts so that these people will be able to provide appealing products and menus that help employees and other consumers meet dietary recommendations. Voluntary, short-term technical assistance will not be sufficient. Rather, long-term innovations in service, education, and surveillance are likely to be required. Quality assurance programs for foods purchased by governments should be adapted whenever possible to include standards consistent with the principles of dietary recommendations.

ACTION 6: *Department secretaries should encourage government employees to consume diets that meet dietary recommendations.*
Department secretaries have initiated programs to promote fitness and discourage smoking in their departments. It is entirely fitting that similar programs encouraging employees to eat in accord with dietary recommendations be initiated together with educational programs to assist them in learning how to accomplish this goal.

ACTION 7: *The U.S. government personnel ultimately responsible for funding official meal functions should offer meals that are consistent with the principles of dietary recommendations.*
This recommendation is applicable to all branches of governments (executive, legislative, and judicial) at all levels (federal, state, and local).

STRATEGY 5: Develop a comprehensive research, monitoring, and evaluation plan to achieve a better understanding of the factors that motivate people to modify their eating habits and to monitor the progress toward implementation of dietary recommendations.

ACTION 1: *The secretaries of USDA and DHHS should mandate increased amounts of intramural research that relate to implementation of dietary recommendations and give high priority to the funding of extramural research in this area.*
Governments as well as the private sector, foundations, and voluntary organizations can perform or fund research that will expedite the implementation of dietary recommendations and surveys that will monitor the progress of implementation and evaluate its impact. Such research would include intervention studies to further understanding of the potential for chronic disease reduction (DHHS, 1988a; NRC, 1989a), social and behavioral studies to elucidate factors that motivate people to modify their food habits over the long term, and tech-

niques to enhance the availability of foods that help people to meet dietary recommendations. A discussion of directions for future research is provided in Chapter 9.

ACTION 2: *Improve the National Nutrition Monitoring System and provide it with adequate resources.*
The National Nutrition Monitoring System consists of a diverse set of surveys and surveillance activities conducted by 12 agencies within six federal departments—DHHS, USDA, DVA, DOD, Commerce, and Labor (DHHS/USDA, 1986, 1989). It provides data on the per-capita availability of foods and nutrients; household and individual food intakes; prevalence of under- and overnutrition using anthropometric, biochemical, and hematological indicators of nutritional status; prevalence of chronic diseases and risk factors for those diseases; and mortality. However, different program obligations and logistical requirements have led to differences in the methods used to collect and present the information (DHHS/USDA, 1989). Budget constraints have led to delays in the start of some surveys and to cuts in the sample sizes. Some groups are frequently excluded from surveys of the civilian noninstitutionalized population, including active-duty military, Native Americans, and people without fixed addresses (including the homeless and migrant families who might have limited access to food [Nestle, 1990]). Other groups, such as racial minorities, are not included in sufficient numbers to permit valid estimates of their nutritional status or health (DHHS/USDA, 1986, 1989). Little information is collected about the population's knowledge of and attitudes toward food and its relationship to health. Better information on the status of the population with respect to recommended dietary patterns will help to plan and target interventions, thus maximizing the budget that will be allocated.

REFERENCES

Benton, J., and L.W. Sullivan. 1990. Food labeling; serving sizes. Fed. Reg. 55:29517-29533.
California Legislature. 1989. Assembly Bill No. 2109. California Legislature—1989-90 Regular Session. 4 pp.
Chipman, H., and P.A. Kendall. 1989. 20 Years of EFNEP: changes and challenges. J. Nutr. Educ. 21:265-269.
Citizens Commission on School Nutrition. 1990. White Paper on School-Lunch Nutrition. Center for Science in the Public Interest, Washington, D.C. 19 pp.
Clarke, G., and J.W. Wise. 1988. USDA adopts "select" beef grade name. Natl. Food. Rev. 11(1):26-27.
Cleveland, L.E., and R.L. Kerr. 1988. Development and uses of the USDA food plans. J. Nutr. Educ. 20:232-238.
DHHS (U.S. Department of Health and Human Services). 1988a. The Surgeon General's

Report on Nutrition and Health. DHHS (PHS) Publ. No. 88-50210. Public Health Service, U.S. Department of Health and Human Services. U.S. Government Printing Office, Washington, D.C. 727 pp.

DHHS (U.S. Department of Health and Human Services). 1988b. Surgeon General's Workshop: Health Promotion and Aging. Proceedings. Public Health Service, U.S. Department of Health and Human Services, Washington, D.C. 109 pp.

DHHS (U.S. Department of Health and Human Services). 1989. Promoting Health/Preventing Disease: Year 2000 Objectives for the Nation. Draft for Public Review and Comment. Office of the Assistant Secretary for Health, Office of Disease Prevention and Health Promotion, Public Health Service. U.S. Department of Health and Human Services, Washington, D.C. 500 pp.

DHHS (U.S. Department of Health and Human Services). 1990a. Healthy People 2000: National Health Promotion and Disease Prevention Objectives. Conference edition. Public Health Service, U.S. Department of Health and Human Services. U.S. Government Printing Office, Washington, D.C. 672 pp.

DHHS (U.S. Department of Health and Human Services). 1990b. Prevention '89/'90: Federal Programs and Progress. Public Health Service, U.S. Department of Health and Human Services. U.S. Government Printing Office, Washington, D.C. 192 pp.

DHHS/USDA (U.S. Department of Health and Human Services/U.S. Department of Agriculture). 1986. Nutrition Monitoring in the United States: A Progress Report from the Joint Nutrition Monitoring Evaluation Committee. DHHS Publ. No. (PHS) 86-1255. U.S. Government Printing Office, Washington, D.C. 356 pp.

DHHS/USDA (U.S. Department of Health and Human Services/U.S. Department of Agriculture). 1989. Nutrition Monitoring in the United States: An Update Report on Nutrition Monitoring. DHHS Publ. No. (PHS) 89-1255. U.S. Government Printing Office, Washington, D.C. 400 pp.

DVA (U.S. Department of Veterans Affairs). 1989. Medical Programs, Fiscal Year 1990. Vol. 11. U.S. Department of Veterans Affairs, Washington, D.C.

Food Chemical News. 1990. Low-fat foods must comply with standards, Shank says. Food Chem. News 32(17):3-4.

GAO (U.S. General Accounting Office). 1989. Food Assistance Programs: Nutritional Adequacy of Primary Food Programs on Four Indian Reservations. Report No. GAO/RCED-89-177. U.S. General Accounting Office, Washington, D.C. 68 pp.

GAO (U.S. General Accounting Office). 1990. Food Assistance Programs: Recipient and Expert Views on Food Assistance at Four Indian Reservations. Report No. GAO/RCED-90-152. U.S. General Accounting Office, Washington, D.C. 63 pp.

Gray, G.E. 1986. Diet, crime and delinquency: a critique. Nutr. Rev. Suppl. 44:89-93.

Hinton, A.W., J. Heimindinger, and S.B. Foerster. 1990. Position of the American Dietetic Association: domestic hunger and inadequate access to food. J. Am. Diet. Assoc. 90:1437-1441.

IOM (Institute of Medicine). 1990. Nutrition Labeling: Issues and Directions for the 1990s. Report of the Committee on the Nutrition Components of Food Labeling, Food and Nutrition Board. National Academy Press, Washington, D.C. 355 pp.

Morris, P.M. 1990. What's for Lunch? II. A 1990 Survey of Options in the School Lunch Program. Public Voice for Food and Health Policy, Washington, D.C. 31 pp.

NCEP (National Cholesterol Education Program). 1990. Report of the Expert Panel on Population Strategies for Blood Cholesterol Reduction. NIH Publication No. 90-3046. National Heart, Lung, and Blood Institute, National Institutes of Health, U.S. Department of Health and Human Services. 139 pp.

NCI/NHLBI (National Cancer Institute/National Heart, Lung, and Blood Institute). 1988. Eating for Life. NIH Publ. No. 88-3000. U.S. Government Printing Office, Washington, D.C. 23 pp.

Nestle, M. 1990. National nutrition monitoring policy: the continuing need for legislative intervention. J. Nutr. Educ. 22:141-144.

NDC (National Dairy Council). 1989. Final Report: The Bridge Project. Translation of Nutrition Research Information into Marketing Strategies for the Dairy Industry. National Dairy Council, Rosemont, Ill. 56 pp.

NIH (National Institutes of Health). 1989. Program in Biomedical and Behavioral Nutrition Research and Training, Fiscal Year 1988. NIH Publ. No. 89-2092. National Institutes of Health, Bethesda, Md. 120 pp.

NRC (National Research Council). 1988. Designing Foods: Animal Product Options in the Marketplace. Report of the Committee on Technological Options to Improve the Nutritional Attributes of Animal Products, Board on Agriculture. National Academy Press, Washington, D.C. 367 pp.

NRC (National Research Council). 1989a. Diet and Health: Implications for Reducing Chronic Disease Risk. Report of the Committee on Diet and Health, Food and Nutrition Board, Commission on Life Sciences. National Academy Press, Washington, D.C. 749 pp.

NRC (National Research Council). 1989b. Recommended Dietary Allowances, 10th edition. Report of the Subcommittee on the Tenth Edition of the RDAs, Food and Nutrition Board, Commission on Life Sciences. National Academy Press, Washington, D.C. 284 pp.

Roberts-Gray, C. 1987. Performance of the Texas Nutrition Education and Training (NET) Program: October 1986 through September 1987. Texas Department of Human Services, Austin, Tex. 120 pp.

Shotland, J. 1989. What's for Lunch? A Progress Report on Reducing Fat in the School Lunch Program. Public Voice for Food and Health Policy, Washington, D.C. 35 pp.

U.S. Army. 1989. Dietary Assessment of U.S. Army Basic Trainees at Fort Jackson, SC. Report No. T6-89. Medical Research & Development Command, U.S. Army Research Institute of Environmental Medicine, Natick, Mass. 301 pp.

U.S. Congress, House. 1989a. Child Nutrition Programs: Issues for the 101st Congress. Serial No. 100-CC. Subcommittee on Elementary, Secondary, and Vocational Education of the Committee on Education and Labor, U.S. House of Representatives. U.S. Government Printing Office, Washington, D.C. 220 pp.

U.S. Congress, House. 1989b. Nutrition Monitoring. Joint hearing before the Committee on Agriculture and the Committee on Science, Space, and Technology, U.S. House of Representatives. Serial No. 101-29. U.S. Government Printing Office, Washington, D.C. 329 pp.

U.S. Congress, House. 1990. Food and Agricultural Resources Act of 1990. Report 101-569, Part 1. Committee on Agriculture, U.S. House of Representatives. U.S. Government Printing Office, Washington, D.C. 914 pp.

U.S. Congress, Senate. 1990. Food, Agriculture, Conservation, and Trade Act of 1990. Report 101-357. Committee on Agriculture, Nutrition, and Forestry, U.S. Senate. U.S. Government Printing Office, Washington, D.C. 1,282 pp.

USDA (U.S. Department of Agriculture). 1981. Eating for Better Health. Program Aid No. 1290. Food and Nutrition Service, U.S. Department of Agriculture, Alexandria, Va. 27 pp.

USDA (U.S. Department of Agriculture). 1983. Menu Planning Guide for School Food Service. Program Aid No. 1260. Food and Nutrition Service, U.S. Department of Agriculture. U.S. Government Printing Office, Washington, D.C. 97 pp.

USDA (U.S. Department of Agriculture). 1984. Make Your Food Dollars Count. Program Aid No. 1344-1347. U.S. Department of Agriculture, Washington, D.C.

USDA (U.S. Department of Agriculture). 1986a. Dietary Guidance Working Group: history and purpose. August. Photocopy. 1 p.

USDA (U.S. Department of Agriculture). 1986b. Make Your Food Dollars Count. Program Aid No. 1385-1388. U.S. Department of Agriculture, Washington, D.C.

USDA (U.S. Department of Agriculture). 1986c. Nutrition and Your Health: Dietary Guidelines for Americans. Home and Garden Bulletin Nos. 232-1 through 232-7. Human Nutrition Information Service, U.S. Department of Agriculture, Hyattsville, Md.

USDA (U.S. Department of Agriculture). 1986d. USDA Comprehensive Plan for a National Food and Human Nutrition Research and Education Program: A Report to Congress. U.S. Department of Agriculture, Washington, D.C. 91 pp.

USDA (U.S. Department of Agriculture). 1987. 1987 Report on USDA Human Nutrition Research and Education Activities. A Report to Congress. U.S. Department of Agriculture, Beltsville, Md. 52 pp.

USDA (U.S. Department of Agriculture). 1988a. Dietary Guidelines and Your Diet: Home Economics Teacher's Guide. Miscellaneous Publ. No. 1457. Human Nutrition Information Service, U.S. Department of Agriculture, Hyattsville, Md. 44 pp.

USDA (U.S. Department of Agriculture). 1988b. 1988 Report on USDA Human Nutrition Research and Education Activities. A Report to Congress. U.S. Department of Agriculture, Beltsville, Md. 68 pp.

USDA (U.S. Department of Agriculture). 1989a. Dietary Guidelines and Your Diet. Home and Garden Bulletin Nos. 232-8 through 232-11. Human Nutrition Information Service, U.S. Department of Agriculture, Hyattsville, Md.

USDA (U.S. Department of Agriculture). 1989b. What is the role of USDA commodity foods in the NSLP? Photocopy. 2 pp.

USDA/DHHS (U.S. Department of Agriculture/U.S. Department of Health and Human Services). 1980. Nutrition and Your Health. Dietary Guidelines for Americans. Home and Garden Bulletin No. 228. U.S. Department of Agriculture/U.S. Department of Health and Human Services, Washington, D.C. 20 pp.

USDA/DHHS (U.S. Department of Agriculture/U.S. Department of Health and Human Services). 1985. Nutrition and Your Health. Dietary Guidelines for Americans, 2nd ed. Home and Garden Bulletin No. 232. U.S. Department of Agriculture/U.S. Department of Health and Human Services, Washington, D.C. 24 pp.

USDA/DHHS (U.S. Department of Agriculture/U.S. Department of Health and Human Services). 1990. Nutrition and Your Health: Dietary Guidelines for Americans, 3rd ed. Home and Garden Bulletin No. 232. U.S. Department of Agriculture/U.S. Department of Health and Human Services, Washington, D.C. 28 pp.

White House. 1970. White House Conference on Food, Nutrition and Health: Final Report. U.S. Government Printing Office, Washington, D.C. 341 pp.

6

Private Sector: Strategies and Actions for Implementation

M EMBERS OF THE private sector must play a large role in helping consumers select more health-promoting foods. They are presented with both opportunities and challenges by the scientific consensus that specific changes in eating habits are likely to reduce substantially the public's risk of heart disease, cancer, and many other diet-related chronic diseases. Food labels and consumer information programs as well as specific product formulations and promotions need to be examined creatively with this in mind.

For the purposes of this report, the private sector is defined broadly as including producers of several major commodities (fruits and vegetables, grains and legumes, dairy products, meat, poultry, fish and seafood, and eggs); food manufacturers and processors and retailers; food service establishments (restaurants, fast-service food establishments, and institutional food-service providers); and work sites (cafeterias and vending machines in office buildings and factories). The private sector is, thus, not a monolith, but a collection of interests often competing for the same consumer dollar. Since any single consumer can eat only a given amount of food each year, the question of who will provide that food becomes a matter of great economic importance.

The entire private sector—from producer to retailer—greatly influences what consumers purchase and consume. In addition, it adapts its products and marketing strategies not only to anticipate and respond to consumer demand but also to create the demand for specific products and services. The committee recognizes that the private sector is in business to sell products and services and make a profit doing so. It therefore recognizes that dietary recommendations will be implemented to the extent that they facilitate, or are not in conflict with, these objectives. The marketer's goal is to sell products, yet implicit in this goal is the responsibility to provide consumers with sufficient product choice and the necessary information to make informed selections.

Many nutrition programs and food products consistent with the principles of dietary recommendations are either already available or under development by the private sector and have been created in response to a growing public interest in health and nutrition. Most of the committee's recommendations in this chapter have already been heard by this societal sector. The committee believes, however, that the various segments of the private sector—supermarkets, food-service establishments, and other purveyors of food—can be encouraged to compete with each other in offering to consumers practical advice on implementing dietary recommendations as well as products developed or modified to be lower in fat, cholesterol, and salt and higher in complex carbohydrates than those currently on the market.

INCENTIVES AND BARRIERS TO IMPLEMENTATION BY THE PRIVATE SECTOR IN GENERAL

Important incentives and barriers that apply to the private sector across the board are discussed below.

Incentives

Competitive Advantage

It is common, although technically inaccurate, to speak of the food industry as though it were monolithic. In reality, as discussed earlier, it is a heterogeneous collection of private-sector entities that compete for a share of the market for similar or related food product lines. It seems increasingly likely that a company will gain a competitive advantage by introducing nutritionally desirable and appealing products that meet the public's growing interest in purchasing health-promoting foods. Consumers are likely to purchase good quality products that help them to meet dietary recommendations as they become more informed and as the organoleptic properties (e.g., taste, odor, mouthfeel, and color) of health-promoting foods and the convenience of their preparation are perceived to improve. According to a national survey conducted by the Food Marketing Institute (FMI) in January 1990, 97% of respondents reported that nutrition is "very" or "somewhat important" to them when they shop for food; 90% reported that they and their families pay at least some attention to the nutritional content of what they eat; and 40% reported that fat content is the nutritional attribute of food to which they pay the most attention (FMI, 1990).

Consumer Confidence

Manufacturers and companies that offer nutritionally desirable foods, products that have complete nutrition labeling, or other useful nutrition information will likely increase customer satisfaction and confidence in their products, thus increasing their sales through new and repeat business. Well-informed customers are generally confident in their product choices and loyal to products recognized as health promoting.

Enhanced Image and Credibility

Image and credibility are very important to all companies. Companies that offer to their customers nutrition information programs as well as health-promoting products, and that market them as such, would be perceived positively by consumers seeking to improve their diets. Positive word-of-mouth advertising by health-care professionals, community organizations, consumer groups, and individual consumers can be as effective as paid advertising in contributing to a company's image.

Cost Reduction and Improved Programs Through Cooperative Efforts

Cooperation and collaboration in implementing dietary recommendations among the private sector, government agencies, health-care professionals, consumer and voluntary organizations, and academia are to be encouraged. This would reduce redundancy, and thus the costs of implementation programs, and would increase their quality by drawing on the combined expertise of those who are part of these various sectors.

Barriers

Restrictive, Confusing, or Nonexistent Government Standards

Some government standards of identity may limit or prohibit the development of new or modified products that are lower in fat, cholesterol, and sodium. Thus, changes in these and in federal or state regulations will be necessary if more nutritionally desirable products with easily recognizable names are to be manufactured. In addition, the lack of uniform definitions for descriptors on food product labels such as *low fat, low cholesterol,* or *lite* creates confusion among consumers and in the private sector itself (IOM, 1990; NRC, 1988).

Inadequate Federal Guidance on Health Claims

The lack of specific federal guidance creates uncertainty in the private sector about how best to communicate knowledge of the connections between diet and health in relation to individual products, thereby permitting the use of confusing, incomplete, or misleading statements to stimulate consumer purchases of certain products. On February 13, 1990, the Food and Drug Administration (FDA) proposed specific guidelines on health claims (Benson and Sullivan, 1990), but no final rule has been issued as of this writing. Recently enacted food labeling legislation gives FDA clear authority to regulate health claims on foods (Food Chemical News, 1990c,d).

Lack of Guidance on Implementation

The lack of practical guidance on how to implement dietary recommendations limits the private sector's ability to make changes in the food supply. Many companies do not employ registered dietitians or nutritionists to evaluate the nutrient content of foods, to develop high-quality and accurate informational materials on healthy eating, or to prepare the nutrition-related statements for product labels and advertising. Chefs and food-service personnel often do not have sufficient background or training in nutrition or in recipe or menu modification.

Cost of Product Development and Research

Considerable research must be undertaken before a company can reasonably decide whether or not to invest in the development and marketing of a nutritionally desirable product. Financial risk can be minimized by thorough assessments in which the most effective research tools are used.

Consumer Concerns about Food Safety

According to the national survey conducted by FMI in 1990, 20% of respondents reported that they were "somewhat" or "mostly doubtful" that the food in their supermarket is safe (FMI, 1990). Both the private and public sectors are responding to the concerns of this group by continuing to take steps to protect the food supply and enlisting the assistance of food scientists and the nutrition community to inform

the public about issues related to food safety. Specific widely publicized incidents can erode consumers' confidence level regarding the
safety of the food supply, but it appears to rebound to initial levels
rather quickly. In April 1989, for example, consumer confidence dropped
to 73% as a result of media reports about contaminated imported
grapes and the use of pesticides and growth regulators in produce.
By January 1990, the level of consumer confidence had rebounded
back to 79% (FMI, 1990).

STRATEGIES AND ACTIONS FOR THE PRIVATE SECTOR

Two general strategies, each of which consists of three actions, are
proposed for the private sector. The first strategy focuses on providing
consumers with information on how to improve their dietary patterns
and motivating them to do so, while the second concerns the production, manufacture, and marketing of nutritionally desirable foods.

**STRATEGY 1: Promote dietary recommendations and
motivate consumers to use them in selecting and preparing foods and in developing healthful dietary patterns.**

ACTION 1: *Make consumers aware of dietary recommendations
and their importance and how available products and services
can be used to meet them.*

Advertising, public relations, and special promotions can inform
consumers about dietary recommendations and thereby help to develop
markets for health-promoting foods. They can also enhance the reputation
of companies and brand-name products that provide accurate and
practical information to consumers.

The private sector can play a major role in cooperative efforts involving health-care professionals; academicians; consumer, health, and civic
organizations; and governments to develop a variety of consumer information and education programs and materials that would explain ways in
which eating patterns can be adapted to meet dietary recommendations. The programs must emphasize the total diet as well as gradual
changes in eating habits; messages should be simple, balanced, and consistent.
Chapter 4 identifies some of the major dietary principles that should
form the basis of these programs and materials.

Use of the combined expertise of individuals involved in these
joint ventures has already resulted in the development of nutrition
information programs that go beyond what any individual group can
accomplish. An example is the collaborative effort of the Kellogg
Company with the National Cancer Institute to promote increased
consumption of fiber-rich cereals (Freimuth et al., 1988). In addition

to pooling their expertise, the participants should be encouraged to combine their resources, thereby reducing the costs to each.

In advertising and in other consumer materials, health-promoting foods should be displayed together (e.g., vegetables and fruits should be shown with low-fat meats, skinless poultry, seafood, nonfat and low-fat dairy products, and whole grains). This will help consumers to visualize the kinds of foods and menus that are recommended to promote good health. Promotional materials should advocate low-fat cooking techniques such as baking, broiling, poaching, steaming, microwaving, or grilling, rather than frying.

The private sector should be encouraged to develop incentive programs for corporations and businesses to promote nutrition messages responsibly. Special awards programs could be established, for example, to increase the visibility of companies that are judged to promote responsible nutrition messages in effective ways.

ACTION 2: *Contribute to efforts to improve the nutrition labeling of food so that it better assists consumers in making informed, nutritionally desirable food choices.*

It is recognized broadly that nutrition labels on food products can help consumers to design diets that meet dietary recommendations. To be more useful, however, they need to be available on more food products and improved in both content and format. The private sector has been actively involved in seeking a solution to current concerns in several areas. For example, they have distributed information to consumers on how to make use of nutrition labeling. An increasing number of foods—now estimated at approximately 60% of all packaged food products—carry nutrition labeling (IOM, 1990). In addition, consumers have been surveyed by segments of the private sector about their interest in and use of food labels and their suggestions for improved labeling (see, for example, FMI, 1990, and Opinion Research Corporation, 1990). Some segments have also developed position statements and provided comments in response to regulatory and congressional efforts to revise food labeling (IOM, 1990). The private sector should continue these activities and avidly support new labeling regulations as issued. As an example, the National Food Processors Association recently organized the Food Label Education Coalition to help consumers use the new food labels that are developed (Coleman, 1990; NFPA, 1990). The coalition is composed of representatives of government agencies; education, consumer, and health organizations; and the food industry. Another committee of the Food and Nutrition Board has addressed nutrition labeling of foods in depth (IOM, 1990).

ACTION 3: *Provide consumers with information at points of purchase so that they may assess quickly some of the nutrition attributes of specific products and brands.*

According to a national survey of consumers by FMI in 1989, the preferred methods of providing nutrition-related information in stores were, in order of priority, pamphlets, nutrition tags on shelves near food items, recipe cards, and in-store demonstrations or videos; but only 55% of those surveyed responded that supermarkets do an excellent or good job in this respect (FMI, 1989b). It appears that food retailers have an opportunity to improve their performance in this area.

STRATEGY 2: Continue to increase the availability of a wide variety of appealing foods that help consumers to meet dietary recommendations.

ACTION 1: *Develop more nutritionally desirable products that appeal to consumers.*

The private sector has been modifying traditional products as technology permits to make them more nutritionally desirable—usually by reducing their total fat, saturated fat, sodium, or sugar content or by increasing their fiber content. In addition, the private sector is developing an increasing number of nutritionally desirable food products that are appealing. Examples include whole-grain, ready-to-eat cereals with no added sweeteners; low-fat dairy products; fat-free or very-low-fat pastries and baked goods; frozen dinner entrees low in total fat, saturated fat, and sodium; and lower-fat hamburger patties served in fast-service food establishments. Of course, each food need not meet specific target levels specified in dietary recommendations (e.g., 30% or less of calories from fat; see chapter 4). Nevertheless, consumers are more likely to meet these recommendations if their diets are composed largely of nutritionally desirable products.

ACTION 2: *Contribute to efforts to revise, or develop as appropriate, food-quality criteria (such as standards of identity and grading), pricing structures, and food product descriptors to promote the production of more nutritionally desirable food products.*

Standards of identity developed by the government specify mandatory ingredients for many common foods such as catsup, cheese, ice cream, frankfurters, bread, and mayonnaise. These standards have helped to ensure the quality and consistency of products by prohibiting manufacturers from substituting less expensive ingredients. Food products that deviate from these standards (e.g., ice cream with less fat than specified) must be renamed in most cases (e.g., frozen dessert) or labeled as imitation (e.g., imitation ice cream). Thus, standards of identity can inhibit the replacement of high-fat or high-cholesterol components of foods with nonfat or low-fat ingredients. They should be updated whenever possible to promote the production of more nutritionally desirable versions of food products. The FDA is allowing the test marketing of several products that deviate from their standards of identity but still carry their traditional names (e.g., nonfat cottage cheese [Shank, 1990a], light eggnog [Shank, 1990b], lowfat ice cream [Food Chemical News, 1990b], and light sour cream [Food Chemical News, 1990a]) to measure consumer acceptance.

The carcasses of red meat animals are graded to indicate the quality of table meats. Yet the current U.S. grading system, which is basic to the marketing and pricing of red meat, deters the production of lean meat by linking quality grades to fat content. The nomenclature is not identical for beef, pork, and lamb, but generally, the higher the fat content of the muscles (marbling), the higher the quality grade, since marbling improves the chances of the meat being flavorful, juicy, and tender when cooked (NRC, 1988). Prime and Choice are the two highest grades, but most meat sold is Choice and Select. A marketing system that promoted the leaner grades, primarily Select, would increase the availability of lower-fat meats, which consumers say they want (Sweeten et al., 1990).

ACTION 3: *Engage in practices leading to the greater availability of nutritionally desirable products that will assist consumers in meeting dietary recommendations.*

The private sector should fund and conduct research on nutritional attributes of products as well as on consumer attitudes, knowledge, and practices for ideas to provide consumers with products they want and need. They should also conduct marketing and informational campaigns to increase consumption of health-promoting products. It is important that this research be wide-ranging and help commodity producers, manufacturers, processors, retailers, and food-service establishments learn how to improve their products and their promotional campaigns. This information should be shared throughout the private sector, including supermarkets and the media, as well as with health-care professionals.

STRATEGIES AND ACTIONS APPLIED TO SPECIFIC SEGMENTS OF THE PRIVATE SECTOR

Fruits and Vegetables (Produce)

The committee recommends that the produce industry implement a national fruit and vegetable campaign based on social marketing approaches with extensive use of the media to promote consumption of five or more servings of fruits and vegetables daily as a goal to be reached by the year 2000. The goal should be to increase consumer awareness of the health benefits of fruits and vegetables; to motivate people to eat more of them while emphasizing their convenience, taste, great variety, and relatively low costs; and to provide tips on how to incorporate at least five servings of these foods into the diet each day. Successful implementation of this campaign will require leadership and coordination from both the Produce Marketing Association and the United Fresh Fruit and Vegetable Association; large commodity producer groups and fruit and vegetable corporations; and leaders from the food industry, public health agencies, and voluntary health organizations.

There is precedent for such a campaign. In 1988, the fruit and vegetable industry, in cooperation with the California Department of Health Services and the California Department of Food and Agriculture, began a 3-year statewide campaign to promote the consumption of five servings of fruits and vegetables per person per day and at least 500 lbs of produce per person per year by the year 2000 (Foerster and Bal, 1990). This California initiative, entitled "5 A Day—For Better Health," has been very successful in generating positive media coverage and encouraging the participation of supermarkets and other segments of the produce industry in promoting and implementing the campaign.

The creation of a national, federally mandated research and promotion program for all produce would provide a mechanism for raising funds from growers and the produce industry to enhance the positive image of fruits and vegetables through paid advertising and would ensure the necessary cooperation among the produce industry (especially the leading producers), its trade associations, and the U.S. Department of Agriculture (USDA). In the past, promotion programs for beef, milk, watermelon, and potatoes have led to increased sales (Hitt, 1977; Mayer, 1990).

The produce industry should promote and support government efforts to develop innovative programs that will help low-income families attain greater access to fruits and vegetables. For example, 10 states have received federal funds as part of a demonstration project to provide participants in the Special Supplemental Food Program for Women, Infants, and Children (the WIC program) with coupons that can be used to purchase fresh fruits and vegetables at local farmers markets (U.S. Congress, 1988; USDA, 1990). If implemented more broadly, this program could increase the consumption of fruits and vegetables by those with economic limitations.

Some consumers are concerned about residues of pesticides on some foods (FMI, 1990), and may therefore be reticent to eat more fruits and vegetables. The produce industry should promote the message that the health benefits of produce outweigh any possible negative effects from pesticides or other residues. The food industry is responding to consumers' pesticide fears in several ways, for example, public education about the safety and benefits of pesticides and efforts in the agricultural sector to reduce their use (Ravenswaay, 1989).

Grains and Legumes

Consumption of grain products in the United States has increased over the past two decades. This has been in forms that include cereals, pastas, and baked goods. The formulation of grain food products involves millers, wholesale bakeries, food processors, cereal manufacturers, and food retailers with their in-store bakeries. The number of in-store bakeries grew from 18,850 in 1987 (Boisisio et al., 1990) to an estimated 23,007 in 1990 (Malovany, 1990). Wholesale bakers are producing more varieties of bread and reformulating their products to contain less-saturated fats and oils (Malovany, 1990). The committee encourages the baking industry to expand its output of whole-grain and lower-fat products, such as whole-grain, low-fat breads, rolls, bagels, pitas, and pastas, and baked rather than fried grain-based snacks, such as corn chips.

Consumption of legumes (i.e., dried beans and peas; see Chapter 4) increased from 6.9 lbs per capita in 1970 to 8.3 lbs in 1987 (Putnam, 1989). Producer-supported organizations such as the American Dry Bean Board and the USA Dry Pea & Lentil Industry have developed promotional materials that include product information and recipe ideas for use by food editors in the media, food and nutrition professionals, restaurants, and consumers in an effort to increase consumption of legumes. Budget constraints limit the scope and reach of these promotional initiatives (Dry Pea & Lentil News, 1990; Hays, 1990).

In light of the dietary recommendation to increase consumption of grains (particularly whole grains) and legumes, both industries should consider a campaign similar to that recommended for the produce industry to encourage consumption of these products. Since these segments of the private sector are relatively fragmented, such campaigns should include regional components and other efforts applicable to the similarly dispersed fish and seafood industry. Both should begin to promote dietary recommendations to encourage consumption of their products.

Dairy

The dairy industry and companies that sell dairy foods should promote more aggressively nonfat and low-fat dairy products and explain to consumers the differences in their fat and calorie contents. In the committee's judgment, the industry has not promoted adequately these products in its advertising and educational materials, nor in some cases has it made them widely available. For example, consumers in California did not have 1% fat milk in the marketplace until January 1990 (CMAB, 1990; Times Delta, 1990). At that time, however, the California Milk Advisory Board made a commendable effort to educate consumers by comparing the nutrient contents of fresh milk with different levels of fat.

The committee concluded, after discussion with several dairy economists, that one of the major barriers to promoting nonfat and low-fat dairy products may be an unwillingness by some segments of the dairy industry to imply that their full-fat product line (whole milk, cheese, butter, and ice cream)—the focus of their traditional image—may be less nutritionally desirable. The impetus for making changes has evolved from recognition of the need to reduce the fat content of dairy products to take advantage of consumers' increasing interest in diet and health. A recent report commissioned by the National Dairy Council suggested that it would be "self-defeating" for the dairy industry to continue to "ignore" or "fight" the growing scientific consensus on reducing dietary fat (NDC, 1989, p. 5). This industry should work with voluntary health and professional organizations to develop consumer education materials that promote the consumption of a variety of nonfat and low-fat dairy products that help people to meet dietary recommendations.

The committee believes that dietary recommendations and national campaigns to encourage the U.S. population to reduce substantially its dietary fat intake should be perceived by the dairy industry as an opportunity rather than as a threat, since many low-fat products are available. These include low-fat (and, in some cases, fat-free) milk, cheese, yogurt, ice cream, and sour cream.

The committee encourages the dairy industry to work toward changing the milk pricing system to encourage dairy producers to breed, feed, and manage their herds for production of lower-fat milk in accordance with changing consumer demands. Joint initiative, willingness, and action by the dairy industry and USDA will be required to change the current price support system for dairy products. Admittedly, a change that reduces the price for the butterfat component of the milk will penalize dairy farmers whose cows produce milk with a high butterfat content and may increase the cost of low-fat dairy products to consumers (NDC, 1989).

In addition, the dairy industry should work with the FDA to redefine low-fat milk as 1% milk. Currently, 2% milk does not meet FDA's working definition (which carries no legal weight) of a low-fat food, which FDA defines as a food that contains no more than 2 g of fat per serving (IOM, 1990). Since 2% milk contains 5 g of fat per serving, it seems inaccurate and perhaps even deceptive to label 2% milk as low-fat, especially since consumers drink more of it than any other type of milk. Changing the standard and nomenclature as recommended will send a strong economic signal to dairy producers that dairy animals should be fed and managed in ways that inhibit excess fat production. In addition, efforts should be accelerated to enhance the appeal, and thereby the acceptance, of 1% and skim (nonfat) milk. States could require, for example, that a specified quantity of these milks be fortified with nonfat milk solids to increase their taste appeal.

Meat

The meat industry has been responding to consumer demands for leaner meat. The pork and beef industries have conducted research and allocated resources to implement technologies to reduce subcutaneous (below the skin) and intramuscular fat levels and thus produce leaner animals. Further changes in feeding, breeding, and selection by all producers are needed to accelerate the trend toward leaner animals. In setting realistic goals for such changes, industry must consider consumer acceptance of the palatability of meat products (Sweeten et al., 1990). Economic, marketing, and research policies should be redefined to encourage not only the production of leaner animals but also the processing of low-fat animal products and to discourage the reintroduction of trimmed fat at another point in the food chain (e.g., using beef tallow to cook french fries in fast-service food establishments).

The meat industry should continue to work with USDA to develop a grading system that provides economic rewards for leaner meat. In 1972, Canada changed its beef grading system to counter the economic bias toward fat (NRC, 1988). Since the grading change, in which lean meat receives the highest grades, the Canadian market has become dominated by lean beef, which now commands the premium price. A modification of Canada's grading system may be a model to consider in the United States. In 1988, the U.S. grading system was modified to allow the renaming of U.S. Good to U.S. Select (NRC, 1988). This name change provided the industry with an opportunity, through the use of a more positive grade name, to improve its marketing of beef with less marbling than that in Prime or Choice.

One incentive for meat producers to change their current production practices would be to pay them on the basis of trim weight rather than on a fat-in-carcass weight. If subcutaneous fat were removed from the carcass immediately after slaughter (hot-fat trimming), the price would be based on the trimmed carcass, in effect penalizing the producer for additional fat. At present, however, carcasses trimmed immediately after slaughter are ineligible for quality grading since they cannot be accurately graded for yield (NRC, 1988).

The meat industry should also work with USDA to adopt a national uniform standard for the fat content of ground beef. USDA has defined *lean* and *extra lean* meat as containing no more than 10 and 5% by weight, respectively, for all meats except ground beef (IOM, 1990)—the most frequently consumed form of beef in the United States (Block et al., 1985). Since there is no federal definition of lean ground beef, individual states and supermarkets have set their own standards (Liebman, 1988). Thus, it is difficult for consumers to ascertain from the labels the level of fat in the ground beef products they purchase. It may not be possible to extend the 10 and 5% definitions of *lean* and *extra lean* to ground beef, but national definitions and standards should be set.

The committee also recommends that the meat industry adopt and promote a consistent policy of trimming the exterior fat on meat in retail grocery stores to a thickness of 1/4 in. or less. The rationale, benefits, and techniques for accomplishing this should be shared with supermarket chains around the United States. The industry should continue to promote consumption of 3-oz portions of cooked lean, trimmed meat prepared by nonfat or low-fat cooking methods in its advertising, public relations, and consumer education materials. Many consumers will need to be informed that 3-oz portions are smaller than those typically consumed in the United States.

Processed meat products (e.g., luncheon meats and frankfurters) often contain high levels of fat and sodium, which can and should be reduced. Such changes would enable the meat products industry to recapture the segment of the consumer market that no longer purchases these products. Several low-fat and low-sodium versions of these products have become available; more should be offered. Niche marketing could establish small markets (beachheads) that could grow when increased consumer awareness makes such products popular.

Poultry

The traditional U.S. diet contains more poultry—chicken, turkey, duck, and goose—than ever before (Bishop and Christensen, 1989;

see also Chapter 3), partly because of the relatively low price of many poultry products and the public's perception that poultry is lower in calories, fat, and cholesterol. In addition, the poultry industry has developed and introduced many new, easily prepared consumer products—from cut up chickens and prepackaged parts to boneless and skinless breasts. Chicken products have also proliferated at many fast-service food establishments; several chains have made them center-pieces of their menus (Bishop and Christensen, 1989). In its advertising, public relations, and information materials, the poultry industry should encourage consumers to prepare poultry by means other than frying, to remove the skin and any subcutaneous fat before eating, and to serve 3-oz cooked portions along with other low-fat foods.

Like the meat industry, the poultry industry should continue to modify breeding and feeding methods to produce animals with less fat. The current practice of selecting strains for leanness and for improved feed efficiency not only helps to reduce the fat content of the bird but also improves its growth and increases carcass yield (NRC, 1988). A report by the Board on Agriculture of the National Research Council (NRC, 1988) suggests that leaner poultry products can be produced by manipulating the nutrient content of the feed and by marketing younger broilers—a practice now being undertaken.

The committee recommends that the poultry industry work with USDA to develop a uniform standard for the amount of fat in ground turkey, a product that is usually lower in fat than even extra-lean ground beef or pork. However, in the absence of a federal standard (and, frequently, state standards), manufacturers develop their own definitions. Although most brands are relatively lean, ranging from 7 to 14% fat by weight (Giant Food, Inc., 1988), the committee believes that USDA should define lean and extra lean ground turkey as well as beef.

Processed poultry products, including luncheon meats and frankfurters, are typically lower in fat than are similar products made from red meats. However, many are still high in fat and contain high levels of sodium (NRC, 1988). Given the convenience and ready availability of these products, the committee recommends that the poultry industry take further initiatives to reduce the fat and sodium contents of its processed products as much as possible without unnecessarily sacrificing taste and quality.

Fish and Seafood

The National Fish and Seafood Promotional Council, established by the U.S. Department of Commerce in 1986, was the first national generic advertising and public relations program to promote the nutritional benefits of fish and seafood products to consumers. The activities of this congressionally established group of industry representatives are important in developing a coordinated message to consumers from this fragmented industry composed primarily of many small producers. The council could be instrumental in increasing per-capita fish and shellfish consumption; at 15.9 lbs per capita per year (edible meat), consumption is at record levels, although this represents little growth since 1986, when per-capita consumption was 14.7 lbs (NMFS, 1988, 1990).

Specific campaigns are needed to support dietary recommendations and the role of fish and seafood in healthful diets. This could be accomplished through cooperative efforts by industry organizations (such as the National Fisheries Institute), the government (such as the National Marine Fisheries Service and the National Institutes of Health), regional seafood marketing groups, health-care professionals, academia, and voluntary and professional organizations (such as the American Heart Association and the American Dietetic Association).

The fish and seafood industry should expand efforts to organize spokespeople to communicate dietary recommendations in a credible fashion. One special opportunity to promote fish and seafood consumption as part of a healthful diet exists during National Seafood Month (October). Consumer information materials developed by the industry should promote fish and seafood on the basis of their good taste, ease of preparation, and nutritional benefits and should explain how these foods relate to dietary recommendations.

Almost 20% of consumers report that they eat more fish as one means to improve their diets (FMI, 1990). Some, however, are concerned about the safety of fish and seafood as a result of highly publicized incidents of fish contaminated with environmental effluents or natural toxins, pollution of coastal waters, and the lack of a mandatory inspection system (Dicks and Harvey, 1989; IOM, 1991). The Food and Nutrition Board recently evaluated the safety of fish and seafood. It reported that while these foods are usually "wholesome and unlikely to cause illness, . . . there are areas of risk," particularly from the consumption of raw clams, oysters, and mussels (IOM, 1991, p. 1). The food industry can help to reduce health risks associated with fish and seafood consumption by taking all appropriate measures to ensure the quality and safety of these products and by informing consumers about proper ways to select and prepare them.

Eggs

Egg consumption has declined steadily over the past several decades (see Chapter 3), partly because of concerns about nutrition and health. In response, the egg industry has developed recipes and promotional material demonstrating the use of eggs in health-promoting recipes and menus that are compatible with (and refer to) the principles of dietary recommendations. It should also inform consumers how to substitute egg whites for whole eggs in various recipes and thus avoid the egg's cholesterol content, which is found in the yolk.

The industry should continue its research and development of new products containing only egg whites. Simplesse, a recently approved fat substitute, is manufactured from protein found in egg white or milk (Morrison, 1990). The egg industry should also conduct research on ways to reduce the cholesterol content of egg yolk and to discover alternative industrial or nonfood uses for this component.

Food Manufacturers and Processors

These industries are developing new products and modifying existing ones to increase the availability of foods that are reduced or low in total fat, saturated fat, cholesterol, and sodium, an activity the committee supports. In addition, they should take opportunities to provide consumers with information on how their products relate to overall dietary recommendations. One route, now in use, is the provision of toll-free 800 telephone numbers on food packages to encourage consumers to call with comments, questions, or requests for written materials. This is an excellent way to provide consumers with information in the form of recipes, preferred food preparation methods, and government brochures explaining dietary recommendations. Information could also be disseminated over 900 telephone numbers, which are toll calls.

These segments of the food industry along with the public sector should support more basic research in several areas, including nutrient retention, food flavors, textures, and preservation. More information in these areas would enable the food industry to produce food products that consumers find acceptable and help them meet dietary recommendations. New product and marketing research is ongoing at most large food companies.

Food manufacturers and processors should refrain from fortifying their products with nutrients in the absence of a demonstrated public health need or in ways that are considered inappropriate by the scientific community or FDA. In recent years, foods appear to be fortified not as a public health measure to ensure adequate intake of various nutrients but as part of marketing strategies to increase sales by suggesting that a product is more nutritious than a similar product of a competitor. When heavily fortified foods are promoted on the basis of their added nutrients, consumers may be misled about what defines a nutritious food or diet. Highly fortified and enriched foods are not required by most people who follow or are attempting to follow dietary recommendations.[1]

Food Retailers

A variety of user-friendly informational programs and materials have been used (and in some cases developed in whole or in part) by food retailers to show consumers how to eat nutritiously in practical, flexible ways (FMI, 1989a). Many supermarkets already provide brochures, videos, store tours conducted by nutritionists, demonstrations of healthful cooking, and toll-free telephone numbers on nutrition-related topics and include information about nutrition in newspaper advertisements as well as in television and radio spots. In addition, supermarkets have developed cooperative projects with the American Heart Association, the American Dietetic Association, local hospitals, universities, and federal agencies and can look for new opportunities to work with nutrition experts to communicate accurate nutrition information. The committee applauds these initiatives and encourages more retailers to participate.

An increasing number of supermarkets in the United States have undertaken shelf-labeling programs that identify products that are low in fat, cholesterol, sodium, calories, or sugar or that are good sources of fiber (FMI, 1989a). Some of them also provide consumer brochures that list the foods by category according to nutrition criteria. These aids not only help customers identify products with nutritionally desirable characteristics but can also increase the sales of some of these products. For example, one study showed that the relative market share of shelf-labeled products increased 4 to 8% over a 2-year period (Levy et al., 1985).

Giant Food, Inc., a Washington, D.C.-based food retailer with stores in both the District of Columbia and nearby Baltimore, Maryland, worked with the National Cancer Institute, the National Heart, Lung, and Blood Institute, and FDA to develop model consumer information programs on diet and cancer, diet and heart disease, and shelf-labeling programs, respectively (Light et al., 1989). Program components included the provision of store bulletins containing information and recipes, media advertising on connections between diet and health, and shelf tags providing nutrition information (e.g., highlighting foods low in sodium or high in fiber). FMI (1989a) has compiled a list and brief description of nutrition information programs in supermarkets across the United States.

One example of a successful collaborative industry-sponsored consumer information program is *Meat Nutri-Facts*, which was developed by FMI, the American Meat Institute, and the National Live Stock and Meat Board in 1985 (FMI/AMI/NLMB, 1985). In 1987, this program was joined by *Poultry Nutri-Facts*, produced by FMI with the National Broiler Council and the National Turkey Federation (FMI/ NBC/NTF, 1987), and in 1988 it was joined by *Seafood Nutri-Facts*, developed by FMI and the National Fisheries Institute (FMI/NFI, 1988). Elements of these programs, which are available in many supermarkets throughout the United States, provide point-of-purchase consumer information, including nutrient and calorie data and recipes, on various products and cuts. This information is conveyed by store signs, recipe cards, brochures, and videos that identify relatively low fat cuts of animal flesh as well as low-fat cooking methods and nutrition information for a 3-oz cooked serving. Information derived from this program is also supplied to the industry and to health-care professionals.

The results of consumer surveys conducted by retailers on the effectiveness of their nutrition information programs should be shared with government agencies and health-related organizations. Supermarket trade associations can also play a key role in evaluating consumer nutrition information programs and disseminating results widely. The committee encourages retailers and their trade associations to go even further by conducting, funding, or collaborating on research to determine consumer attitudes about nutrition, the effectiveness of point-of-purchase nutrition information programs, and topics related to dietary recommendations. This information should be shared throughout the food industry as well as with health organizations, educators, and governments. The FMI annual *Trends* report (FMI, 1990) and its cooperative research studies on nutrition and food trends in conjunction with *Better Homes and Gardens* magazine (FMI/BHG, 1988a,b,c,d, 1989) are two examples of an ongoing effort by the retail food industry to monitor consumer attitudes. Supermarket trade associations should continue to provide their members with information and studies on nutrition issues from a variety of sources.

An increasing number of retailers are preparing their own products in the store (such as salads, entrees, and desserts) and thus can modify the ingredients used and the methods of preparation to reduce fat and sodium. Some of them have their own processing facilities (e.g., a bakery, dairy, ice cream plant, or canning facility). Retailers can use these resources to produce more nutritionally desirable products. They should also ask suppliers of store-brand products to modify the products to make them more nutritionally desirable. In some cases, retailers can develop specifications for items they are willing to purchase. If efforts are made to ensure that the products are appealing, consumer demand for them should increase.

In some parts of the United States (e.g., very small towns, rural areas, and economically deprived areas of cities), people may depend heavily on a small area supermarket or grocery store for their food purchases. The committee believes that these small retailers have a special responsibility to stock as great a variety of health-promoting foods as they are able at reasonable prices to help their patrons meet dietary recommendations.

Food-Service Establishments

The average U.S. consumer eats one of every five meals away from home (Sweet, 1989). The food-service share of a consumer's food dollar has risen from 25% in 1950 (NRA, 1988) to more than 40% in 1987 (NRA, 1989). Thus, food providers (e.g., restaurants, fast-service food establishments, and institutional food-service companies) provide a substantial share of the U.S. diet, and their policies and procedures can have a considerable impact on the foods that are consumed. They can thus have an important role in helping consumers make health-promoting food choices. Their future profits may well depend on how well they accommodate the increasing number of people who wish to eat nutritiously when they eat out (Granzin and Bahn, 1988).

Restaurants, fast-service food establishments, institutional food-service providers, and even caterers have special opportunities and incentives to improve the nutritional quality of their menus and product offerings. For example, they can make available one or more items for each course (e.g., entree and dessert) that are consistent with the principles of dietary recommendations and, in general, initiate changes in food preparation practices to comply with dietary recommendations. Increased customer satisfaction, loyalty, or increased sales provide the major incentive for restaurants to make changes that are consistent with the principles of dietary recommendations. According to a 1986 Gallup Poll, 4 of 10 consumers said they were trying to consume more vegetables and fewer fats, meats, and fried foods when they ate out (NRA, 1990). Fifty-nine percent of respondents in a 1988 poll conducted for the National Restaurant Association (NRA) said they rank nutritious menu items second on a list of 10 features they like to see in a restaurant (Sweet, 1989). At present, approximately 40% of restaurants offer menu items that are reduced in fat, calories, salt, and cholesterol (Sweet, 1989). In mid- and upscale restaurants, health-promoting items account for 15% of all sales (Regan, 1986). Many of the expensive to moderately priced restaurants that have added nutritionally desirable menu items are achieving success, as reflected in increased sales (Framkin, 1988). Experimental pilot projects have shown that the addition of health-promoting items to a menu need not require extensive effort and expense and that they can result in increases in sales (Scott et al., 1979).

Food-service establishments should also accept a social responsibility to make health-promoting foods easily accessible both to those who explicitly seek them and to those who do not. For example, managers could add fresh fruit alternatives to menus or dessert carts so that they would not have to be specially requested. Some nutritionally desirable items may not have sold well in the past simply because diners were unaware that they were available.

Restaurateurs should encourage the NRA to (1) develop a manual with health-promoting alternatives, including specific information on ingredients, preparation, training, costs, and successful introduction in various markets; (2) track and publish the types of health-promoting alternatives that are most popular with consumers; and (3) engage in research on the most effective means of presenting dietary information on menus. In addition, the industry should encourage its trade magazines to carry more stories on dietary recommendations and to provide examples of successful and unsuccessful means of implementation. These actions will help convince restaurant owners and chefs that the adoption of healthful alternatives is feasible and economical and will assist them in determining the best times (primarily in terms of public acceptance) to introduce new items and how to do it. The NRA's *Nutrition Guide for the Restaurateur* (NRA, 1986) is one step that has already been taken in this direction.

Waiters and waitresses should be given basic information about how the restaurant's chefs prepare various dishes so that they can respond knowledgeably to questions asked by consumers trying to follow dietary recommendations. Many food-service establishments may find this recommendation difficult to implement because of frequent staff turnover. The menus themselves could be more descriptive by containing information on how foods are prepared.

In their publicity and advertising, food-service establishments should highlight the availability of menu items that help consumers meet dietary recommendations. This information should also be conveyed to local restaurant reviewers, food editors, and health organizations to inform consumers where nutritionally desirable foods can be obtained. Messages to consumers should focus not only on the health-promoting features of these foods but also on their good taste and appealing presentation.

Restaurants, fast-service food establishments, and food-service providers (e.g., cafeterias at work sites and hospitals), can also help consumers by providing certain information (e.g., total calories, calories from fat, and types of oils used in preparation) on menus or on display cards. Many consumers might be surprised to learn that the salad dressing added to a garden salad at a fast-service food restaurant could supply the same number of calories as a roast beef sandwich and french fries but as much as 50% more fat, depending on the type and amount of dressing used. It is important that consumers know not only the total fat content but also the kind of fat contained in the food. Managers of fast-service food establishments could also display signs notifying consumers that they will prepare items in special ways upon request (e.g., eliminating mayonnaise-based sauces).

Fast-service food restaurants enjoy great popularity. On any day, 20% of the U.S. population is estimated to consume their products; young families with children are most likely to frequent these restaurants (ACSH, 1985), and three in five report they are worried about the nutritional value of such food (Consumer Reports, 1988). The major incentives for making changes in the fast-service food industry are similar to those for table-service restaurants. That is, the major chains may benefit by increasing customer satisfaction, loyalty, and sales. Fast-service food purveyors have less of a problem in implementing changes than table-service restaurants do because their menus are more limited and food preparation is more standardized. There is evidence that health-promoting changes in fast-service food offerings can be successful. For example, the introduction of salads has met with considerable success. At McDonald's, salads account for sales of seven cents of every dollar (Consumer Reports, 1988). Other examples of newly introduced products include skinless grilled or baked chicken in addition to hamburger, lower-fat hamburgers, low-fat or fat-free frozen yogurt in addition to ice cream, and 1% or skim milk instead of 2% or whole milk (NRA, 1990; Sugarman, 1990). Confidence in the success of such changes has led to new initiatives in this industry, such as the development by McDonald's of a prominently displayed listing of the ingredients and nutrient content of its offerings.

Restaurants and other meal providers should move toward 100% vegetable shortening in all frying and should adopt other food preparation methods (e.g., reducing fat and salt content in french fries) to help consumers follow dietary recommendations. For fast-service food chains, specific long-term goals should be set as a matter of company policy. Some have already done so. In 1985, most major fast-service food chains fried with an oil mixture containing beef fat (Jacobson and Fritschner, 1986). They have now shifted to vegetable oil for frying (Food Chemical News, 1990e; Sugarman, 1990).

Representatives of the restaurant industry (e.g., the NRA) and the managers and owners of restaurants should encourage schools that train chefs and cooks to place greater emphasis on dietary recommendations, and they should reward the schools that comply by hiring their graduates. Restaurants could also help to defray (or pay) the costs of tuition for employees who take courses in nutrition and new ways to prepare foods. Meals consistent with the principles of dietary recommendations are not likely to become available in restaurants unless chefs and cooks understand the importance of these recommendations and how to implement them into their food selection and preparation practices.

There are several successful models for this action. For example, the Culinary Institute of America in Hyde Park, New York has incorporated the principles of nutrition into its curriculum and runs a public restaurant specializing in nutritious foods (CIA, 1990). Diners are provided with a computer printout showing the amounts of nutrients in each course and the percentage of their meal that is fat, protein, and carbohydrate. The American Culinary Federation Educational Institute has also incorporated a mandatory nutrition component into its curriculum. Community college and technical schools should also provide nutrition education to those planning to enter the restaurant business.

Approximately 1,800 food-service operations in the United States supply meals to businesses, schools, and other institutions. Among these are a few national companies (e.g., ARA Services and Marriott), which control much of the market. For example, Marriott's InFlite Services (which it sold in late 1989) prepared approximately 150 million meals a year for 150 different airlines (Gibbs, 1989). These large companies currently offer a line of health-promoting food alternatives; for example, ARA Services has developed *Treat Yourself Right*, a nutrition education program that merchandises healthful eating at its contracted facilities (Alice Smitherman of ARA Services, personal communication, 1988).

Food-service companies can do more to sell the benefits of healthful eating to their client companies. Benefits to these companies would include increased sales to employees interested in health-promoting food choices, employees' perception that the company cares about their health, and the potential for savings in medical and other company expenses for employees who eat properly. Nutritionally desirable food items should be incorporated into the regular food-service program, thereby obviating the need for people to make a special effort (e.g., stand in a special line) to obtain them.

Hospitals, voluntary health associations, local health departments and government agencies, and other community-based associations should enlist the help of food-service establishments to (1) develop and advertise health-promoting food alternatives for the community, (2) sponsor seminars for cooks and chefs emphasizing dietary recommendations, and (3) sponsor tastings, food fairs, and contests, awarding and recognizing food-service establishments that support dietary recommendations. Liaisons between restaurant chefs and dietitians also can be successful (Renggli, 1986).

Work Sites

An excellent opportunity for implementing dietary recommendations exists within the business world. Many companies maintain restaurants, cafeterias, snack bars, or vending machines for their employees and provide special meals for meetings, employee recognition events, and other occasions. Through these food-providing activities, they exert an influence on the eating habits of millions of U.S. citizens. Work sites are, therefore, excellent channels for health promotion efforts, including the provision of nutrition services and information (ADA/SNE/DHHS, 1986; Glanz, 1986; see also Chapter 3).

According to a national survey of work-site health promotion activities by the U.S. Department of Health and Human Services in 1985, 66% of work sites with more than 50 employees had at least one health promotion activity (DHHS, 1987). Unfortunately, programs on weight control and general nutrition education were among the activities cited least often (in 15 and 17% of work sites, respectively). Although few work-site health promotion activities have been formally evaluated, most employers reported that program benefits outweighed costs; among the benefits cited in this survey were improved health and productivity among their employees and reduced health-care costs.

Comprehensive health promotion programs have been established at many work sites, although nutrition activities, if present, have been low-cost, low-intensity programs aimed primarily at increasing employee awareness and knowledge (ADA/SNE/DHHS, 1986; DHHS, 1987; Glanz, 1986). Such programs are not designed to facilitate eating behavior changes, even though work sites offer the opportunity for long-term interventions as well as environmental and structural changes that can enhance educational messages and support individual behavior changes. Management might be reluctant to make a long-term commitment of resources to implement comprehensive programs and to contract time with health-care professionals to implement the educational programs, assist in the development of appropriate new policies, and work with the food-service staff to improve the nutritional quality of foods made available to employees.

The committee recommends that corporations provide authoritative information to employees on the relationship of dietary practices to health promotion and disease prevention and promote dietary recommendations. Depending on their size and the resources at their disposal, employers could provide this information to their employees through such means as classes, brown bag seminars, payroll stuffers, newsletter articles, contests, posters, displays, articles in in-house publications, and health-promoting menu offerings in company cafeterias. Corporations should consider offering incentives to employees who modify their dietary practices and consistently make health-promoting food choices, and their executives should serve as models of healthful eating. See Chapter 3 for a further discussion of nutrition education programs at work sites.

Corporations should establish a corporate nutrition policy that confirms the company's commitment to healthy dietary practices consistent with dietary recommendations and specifies that stated standards will be applied to meals served in company food-service operations and at company functions. Small corporations without policies should also provide healthful meals at all opportunities, and those without food-service operations should, at the least, offer more fruits, vegetables, whole grains, and low-fat, low-sodium foods in their vending machines.

NOTE

1. In 1980, FDA published voluntary guidelines for manufacturers to promote the rational fortification of foods (Goyan, 1980). This committee supports those guidelines and encourages manufacturers and processors to comply with them. According to FDA, fortification is appropriate (1) to correct a dietary inadequacy recognized by the scientific community to result in a deficiency disease; (2) to restore nutrient levels to those present in a food before conventional processing and storage; (3) to balance the protein, vitamin, and mineral content of the food in relation to the calories it supplies; and (4) to ensure that a substitute food is nutritionally similar to the traditional food it replaces (NRC, 1989; Quick and Murphy, 1982). FDA does not consider it appropriate to fortify fresh produce; meat, poultry, or fish products; sugars; or snack foods such as candies and carbonated beverages.

REFERENCES

ACSH (American Council on Science and Health). 1985. Fast Food and the American Diet. American Council on Science and Health, Summit, N.J. 34 pp.

ADA/SNE/DHHS (American Dietetic Association/Society for Nutrition Education/ U.S. Department of Health and Human Services). 1986. Worksite Nutrition: A Decision-Maker's Guide. American Dietetic Association, Chicago, Ill. 57 pp.

Benson, J.S., and L.W. Sullivan. 1990. Food labeling; health messages and label statements; reproposed rule. Fed. Reg. 55:5175-5192.

Bishop, R.V., and L.A. Christensen. 1989. America's poultry industry. Natl. Food Rev. 12(1):9-13.

Block, G., C.M. Dresser, A.M. Hartman, and M.D. Carroll. 1985. Nutrient sources in the American diet: quantitative data from the NHANES II survey. Am. J. Public Health 122:27-40.

Boisisio, M., J. DeQuattro, B. Hardin, J.K. Kaplan, D. Senft, and N. Wood. 1990. Wheat, a crop in transition. Agric. Res. 38(9):5-17.

CIA (Culinary Institute of America). 1990. The General Foods Nutrition Center at the Culinary Institute of America. Press releases and miscellaneous materials. Culinary Institute of America, Hyde Park, N.Y.

CMAB (California Milk Advisory Board). 1990. Extra light milk debuts—called "the milk of the 90's." Milk Advisor. Winter, pp. 1, 10.

Coleman, R. 1990. NFPA food label education project & consumer research. Presented at the American Heart Association Meeting, Label Use Project, August 28. Public Communications Office, National Food Processors Association, Washington, D.C.

Consumer Reports. 1988. A survival guide to the greasy kid stuff. Consumer Rep. 53:355-361.

DHHS (U.S. Department of Health and Human Services). 1987. National Survey of Worksite Health Promotion Activities. A Summary. Office of Disease Prevention and Health Promotion, Public Health Service, U.S. Department of Health and Human Services. Office of Disease Prevention and Health Promotion, National Health Information Center, Silver Spring, Md. 51 pp.

Dicks, M.R., and D. Harvey. 1989. Issues behind mandatory seafood inspection. Natl. Food Rev. 12(4):30-33.

Dry Pea & Lentil News. 1990. Domestic marketing materials get facelift. Dry Pea & Lentil News 1(1):1.

FMI (Food Marketing Institute). 1989a. FMI Supermarket Directory, Nutrition & Health Programs, 1989. Consumer Affairs Department, Food Marketing Institute, Washington, D.C. 21 pp.

FMI (Food Marketing Institute). 1989b. Trends: Consumer Attitudes & the Supermarket, 1989. Conducted for Food Marketing Institute by Opinion Research Corporation. The Research Department, Food Marketing Institute, Washington, D.C. 65 pp.

FMI (Food Marketing Institute). 1990. Trends: Consumer Attitudes & the Supermarket, 1990. Conducted for Food Marketing Institute by Opinion Research Corporation. The Research Department, Food Marketing Institute, Washington, D.C. 68 pp.

FMI/AMI/NLMB (Food Marketing Institute/American Meat Institute/National Live Stock and Meat Board). 1985. Meat Nutri-Facts. FMI/AMI/NLMB, Washington, D.C.

FMI/BHG (Food Marketing Institute/Better Homes and Gardens). 1988a. Information Sources, Planning and Purchasing, 1988. Conducted for Food Marketing Institute and Better Homes and Gardens Magazine by Opinion Research Corporation. The Research Department, Food Marketing Institute, Washington, D.C. 16 pp.

FMI/BHG (Food Marketing Institute/Better Homes and Gardens). 1988b. A Study of Food Patterns and Meal Consumption, 1988. Conducted for Food Marketing Institute and Better Homes and Gardens Magazine by Opinion Research Corporation. The Research Department, Food Marketing Institute, Washington, D.C. 16 pp.

FMI/BHG (Food Marketing Institute/Better Homes and Gardens). 1988c. A Study of Nutrition, 1988. Conducted for Food Marketing Institute and Better Homes and Gardens Magazine by Opinion Research Corporation. The Research Department, Food Marketing Institute, Washington, D.C. 16 pp.

FMI/BHG (Food Marketing Institute/Better Homes and Gardens). 1988d. Time, Convenience and Entertaining, 1988. Conducted for Food Marketing Institute and Better Homes and Gardens Magazine by Opinion Research Corporation. The Research Department, Food Marketing Institute, Washington, D.C. 16 pp.

FMI/BHG (Food Marketing Institute/Better Homes and Gardens). 1989. Dinnertime USA, Executive Summary, 1989. Conducted for Food Marketing Institute and Better Homes and Gardens Magazine by Total Research Corporation. The Research Department, Food Marketing Institute, Washington, D.C. 16 pp.

FMI/NBC/NTF (Food Marketing Institute/National Broiler Council/National Turkey Federation). 1987. Poultry Nutri-Facts. FMI/NBC/NTF, Washington, D.C.

FMI/NFI (Food Marketing Institute/National Fisheries Institute). 1988. Seafood Nutri-Facts. FMI/NFI, Washington, D.C.

Foerster, S.B., and D.G. Bal. 1990. California's "5 A Day—For Better Health" campaign. Chronic Dis. Notes Rep. 3(1):7-9.

Food Chemical News. 1990a. Another temporary permit granted for light sour cream. Food Chem. News 32(27):49.

Food Chemical News. 1990b. FDA-ers hope to publish lower fat ice cream document. Food Chem. News 32(30):56.

Food Chemical News. 1990c. Health claims additional re-proposal seen likely. Food Chem. News 32(37):3-6.

Food Chemical News. 1990d. Hutt hits need for FDA clearance of new health messages. Food Chem. News 32(37):43-45.

Food Chemical News. 1990e. Three fast food chains switch to vegetable oils for frying. Food Chem. News 32(22):42-43.

Framkin, P. 1988. Lite and healthy. Restaurant Bus. 87:193-208.

Freimuth, V.S., S.L. Hammond, and J.A. Stein. 1988. Health advertising: prevention for profit. Am. J. Public Health 78:557-561.

Giant Food, Inc. 1988. Eat for Health: Poultry Guide. Form 232 (12/88 CMX). Giant Food, Inc., Landover, Md. 12 pp.

Gibbs, N.R. 1989. You want me to eat this?. Time 133:75-76.

Glanz, K. (ed.). 1986. Nutrition at the worksite. J. Nutr. Ed. 18:S1-S92.

Goyan, J.E. 1980. Nutritional quality of foods; addition of nutrients. Final policy statement of the Food and Drug Administration. Fed. Reg. 45:6314-6324.

Granzin, K.L., and K.D. Bahn. 1988. The role of consumers' attitudes toward nutrition in restaurant patronage. J. Nutr. Ed. 20:56-62.

Hays, S. 1990. The Nebraska Dry Bean Commission; the American Dry Bean Board; American Dry Bean Board Members. August 28, 1990. Photocopies.

Hitt, C. 1977. The potato: something good that's good for you. Case study No. 4-577-093 of the Department of Nutrition, Harvard School of Public Health, and the Harvard Business School. Photocopy. 48 pp.

IOM (Institute of Medicine). 1990. Nutrition Labeling: Issues and Directions for the 1990s. Report of the Committee on the Nutrition Components of Food Labeling, Food and Nutrition Board. National Academy Press, Washington, D.C. 355 pp.

IOM (Institute of Medicine). 1991. Seafood Safety (Prepublication Copy). Report of the Committee on Evaluation of the Safety of Fishery Products, Food and Nutrition Board. National Academy Press, Washington, D.C. 446 pp.

Jacobson, M.F., and S. Fritschner. 1986. The Fast-Food Guide. Workman Publishing, New York. 225 pp.

Levy, A.S., O. Mathews, M. Stephenson, J.E. Tenney, and R.E. Schucker. 1985. The impact of a nutrition information program on food purchases. J. Public Policy Market. 4:1-13.

Liebman, B. 1988. The great ground beef deception. Nutr. Action Healthletter 15(8):8-9.

Light, L., J. Tenney, B. Portnoy, L. Kessler, A.B. Rodgers, B. Patterson, O. Mathews, E. Katz, J.E. Blair, S.K. Evans, and E. Tuckermanty. 1989. Eat for Health: a nutrition and cancer control supermarket intervention. Public Health Rep. 104:443-450.

Malovany, D. 1990. The search for new ideas. Bakery 25(7):44-46.

Mayer, C.E. June 20, 1990. Here's the pitch: From nuts to spuds, Congress helps farmers promote their bounty. Washington Post. E1, E8.

Morrison, R.M. 1990. The market for fat substitutes. Natl. Food Rev. 13(2):24-30.

NDC (National Dairy Council). 1989. Final Report: The Bridge Project. Translation of Nutrition Research Information into Marketing Strategies for the Dairy Industry. National Dairy Council, Rosemont, Ill. 56 pp.

NFPA (National Food Processors Association). August 16, 1990. New coalition to develop nutrition education program. Press release. National Food Processors Association, Washington, D.C.

NMFS (National Marine Fisheries Service). 1988. Fisheries of the United States, 1987. National Oceanic and Atmospheric Administration, U.S. Department of Commerce. U.S. Government Printing Office, Washington, D.C. 116 pp.

NMFS (National Marine Fisheries Service). 1990. Fisheries of the United States, 1989. National Oceanic and Atmospheric Administration, U.S. Department of Commerce. U.S. Government Printing Office, Washington, D.C. 112 pp.

NRA (National Restaurant Association). 1986. A Nutrition Guide for the Restaurateur. National Restaurant Association, Washington, D.C. 72 pp.

NRA (National Restaurant Association). 1988. 1988-1989 Foodservice Industry: National Restaurant Association Pocket Factbook. National Restaurant Association, Washington, D.C. 8 pp.

NRA (National Restaurant Association). 1989. Foodservice Industry: 1987 in Review. National Restaurant Association, Washington, D.C. 8 pp.

NRA (National Restaurant Association). 1990. Nutrition Awareness and the Foodservice Industry: Current Issues Report. National Restaurant Association, Washington, D.C. 20 pp.

NRC (National Research Council). 1988. Designing Foods: Animal Product Options in the Marketplace. Report of the Committee on Technological Options to Improve the Nutritional Attributes of Animal Products, Board on Agriculture. National Academy Press, Washington, D.C. 367 pp.

NRC (National Research Council). 1989. Diet and Health: Implications for Reducing Chronic Disease Risk. Report of the Committee on Diet and Health, Food and Nutrition Board, Commission on Life Sciences. National Academy Press, Washington, D.C. 749 pp.

Opinion Research Corporation. 1990. Food Labeling and Nutrition: What Americans Want. Survey conducted by Opinion Research Corporation for the National Food Processors Association. National Food Processors Association, Washington, D.C. 178 pp.

Putnam, J.J. 1989. Food Consumption, Prices, and Expenditures, 1966-87. Statistical Bulletin No. 773. Economic Research Service, U.S. Department of Agriculture, Washington, D.C. 111 pp.

Quick, J.A., and E.W. Murphy. 1982. The Fortification of Foods: A Review. Agriculture Handbook No. 598. Food Safety and Inspection Service. U.S. Department of Agriculture, Washington, D.C. 39 pp.

Ravenswaay, E.V. 1989. The food industry responds to consumers' pesticide fears. Natl. Food Rev. 12(3):17-20.

Regan, C. 1986. Operators responding to consumer nutrition concerns. Restaurants U.S.A 6:39-41.

Renggli, S. 1986. The Four Seasons Spa Cuisine. Simon and Schuster, New York. 348 pp.

Scott, L.W., J.P. Foreyt, E. Manis, M.P. O'Malley, and A.M. Gotto, Jr. 1979. A low-cholesterol menu in a steak restaurant. J. Am. Diet. Assoc. 74:54-56.

Shank, F.R. 1990a. Cottage cheese deviating from identity standard; temporary permit for market testing. Fed. Reg. 55:32473.

Shank, F.R. 1990b. Eggnog deviating from identity standard; temporary permit for market testing. Fed. Reg. 55:39728-39729.

Sugarman, C. July 31, 1990. Lower-fat fast food: chains feature healthier fare. Washington Post Health. 16.

Sweet, C.A. 1989. Rethinking eating out. FDA Consumer 23:8-13.

Sweeten, M.K., H.R. Cross, G.C. Smith, J.W. Savell, and S.B. Smith. 1990. Lean beef: impetus for lipid modifications. J. Am. Diet. Assoc. 90:87-92.

Times Delta. November 3, 1989. New milk to increase nutrition. Times Delta (Visalia, Calif.).

U.S. Congress. 1988. The Hunger Prevention Act of 1988. Public Law 100-435. U.S. Government Printing Office, Washington, D.C. 35 pp.

USDA (U.S. Department of Agriculture). 1990. Farmers' market coupon demonstration projects, background. Unpublished document.

7

Health-Care Professionals: Strategies and Actions for Implementation

I N THE UNITED STATES, there has been a growing public aware-ness of the role of nutrition in the etiology of many chronic degen-erative diseases and a corresponding demand for information and assistance concerning diet and disease relationships. The U.S. popu-lation looks more and more to health-care professionals to provide clear information confirming this linkage and to establish practical guidelines for dietary regimens that will help to prevent or delay the onset of disease. At the same time, multiple forces, including the need to contain the cost of medical services, may be helping to renew interest among health-care professionals and the public in preventive measures. Good nutrition practices are an essential component of efforts to prevent or control such diseases as atherosclerosis, cancer, hypertension, diabetes, and osteoporosis. Health-care professionals must respond to these increasing needs.

The committee defined health-care professionals as those whose work deals primarily with food and nutrition (e.g., registered dietitians, nutritionists, and nutrition educators); those for whom food and nu-trition issues are important but secondary (e.g., physicians and nurses); and scientists whose basic research concerns the role of food in the etiology of disease. Thus, the target audiences for the implementation strategies and actions proposed in this chapter include nutrition scientists and virtually everyone professionally trained in the delivery of health care.

Increasing expectations that health-care professionals will include nutritional guidance as an integral component of all primary care come at a time when both positive and negative forces are at work. The positive forces include a growing awareness of the escalating social and economic costs of preventable disease and disability, the wide scientific consensus on the nature of dietary recommendations, the increased scope and number of programs in health promotion, and growing evidence of the success of such efforts in reducing nutrition-related risk factors for chronic disease.

The negative forces include inadequate time and lack of compensation to provide the kinds of nutritional guidance that individuals may desire or need, the perception that many people lack interest in eating better and that they do not follow recommended diets, and inadequate knowledge and skills needed to teach people how to improve their diets. A major impediment to implementation of dietary recommendations is the inadequate preparation of health-care professionals (primarily those outside the nutrition field) for these new and expanding roles as promoters of good nutrition and providers of basic information on the subject. Inadequate preparation of many physicians for this role has been recognized for many years (Council on Food and Nutrition, 1963; NRC, 1985).

Fortunately, several voluntary organizations, government agencies, and private associations are attempting to help health-care professionals prepare for their expanded role. Examples include the National Center for Nutrition and Dietetics (ADA, 1990), Project LEAN (Low-Fat Eating for America Now) (Henry J. Kaiser Family Foundation, 1988), the Healthy Mothers, Healthy Babies Public Information Program (DHHS, 1990b), and the national campaigns on cholesterol and high blood pressure education (Cleeman, 1989; Lenfant, 1986; Roccella and Ward, 1984). These and other such programs aim to inform consumers how to improve their dietary practices and to help health-care professionals become better promoters and teachers of nutrition. However, increased coordination and cooperation among such groups and programs are needed to perform this important and complex task effectively.

MULTIPLE ROLES

To implement dietary recommendations, health-care professionals must perform multiple roles, including educational, modeling, organizing, advisory, and investigative roles. Not all these professionals have the same needs for nutrition information to perform each of these roles effectively.

In their *educational* role, health-care professionals may serve as resources on nutrition, food, and health in a variety of ways such as in the preparation of primary and secondary school teachers, the training of health-care professionals (both students and practitioners in classroom settings and in continuing education programs), the motivation and education of individual patients in clinical settings, education of the public, and providing patients with dietary assessments and counseling. Since intellectual acceptance of knowledge by itself rarely fosters lasting change (see Chapter 3), practitioners will need to learn about the forces that govern behavior changes in order to help motivate patients and assist them in acquiring the skills needed to achieve and sustain enduring healthful dietary practices.

By following dietary recommendations themselves, health-care professionals serve as highly credible role models for patients and the public. In this *modeling* role, they can provide information and dietary advice based in part on their personal experiences that may help others to improve their eating habits.

As *organizers*, health-care professionals can initiate or contribute to community programs to improve nutrition. To accomplish this, they may act as individuals or work through professional societies or other health care-related organizations.

The *advisory* role of health-care professionals includes providing legislators and government officials with the information needed to promulgate desirable regulations and guidelines pertaining to food, nutrition, and health policy.

The *investigative* role is carried out primarily by health-care professionals in institutions or organizations involved in basic or applied research. However, community practitioners can play this role as well. As an example, the recognition that contaminated tryptophan supplements may cause serious toxicity was made by a practicing physician (Altman, 1989; CDC, 1989). There is great need for additional insights into the causal relationships between diet, genetic factors, and organic diseases, for more knowledge of the factors that govern behavior change, and for information on how to mobilize communities to promote healthy behaviors. It is certain that there will be additional discoveries in these areas. Thus, current dietary recommendations, which represent the best understanding of nutrition science to date, may need to be revised in the future. (See Chapter 9 for suggested research topics.)

CURRENT STATUS AND FUTURE NEEDS OF SOME HEALTH-CARE PRACTITIONERS

In this section, nutritionists, physicians, nurses, health educators, and other health-care practitioners are described in terms of their roles and needs in implementing dietary recommendations. The ordering of these professional groups does not reflect any hierarchy of importance to their respective and complementary tasks.

Nutritionists

The pool of qualified nutrition personnel needed to implement dietary recommendations is varied. It consists of nutritionists working in a variety of settings, including state and local health departments, community nutrition programs, policy and advocacy organizations, educational institutions at all levels, and research facilities. This pool includes approximately 44,000 registered dietitians (American Dietetic Association, personal communication, 1990), 4,700 public health nutrition personnel (Kaufman, 1989), 2,800 scientists in the American Institute of Nutrition (American Institute of Nutrition, personal communication, 1990), and 270 physicians board certified in nutrition (American Board of Nutrition, personal communication, 1990). Because some nutrition professionals are members of two or more of these categories and some are not included in any of them, the total number involved in this effort will be different from this total.

To deepen the knowledge of nutrition specialists and enhance their skills in teaching a wide variety of publics to base their eating patterns on dietary recommendations, traditional education programs must be improved. For example, curricula must emphasize both the social and behavioral aspects of promoting dietary changes as well as the scientific basis of the recommendations. In addition, curricula should include relevant material from the food and agricultural sciences. This requires a delicate balance. Too much emphasis on the scientific fundamentals could lead to omission of the practical aspects of nutrition and dietary change. Public health and other community-based nutrition specialists who work actively on promoting health among target populations need additional training on how to integrate into their programs the growing evidence on diet and health relationships and how to manage complex community intervention programs.

Registered dietitians and other nutrition specialists must be trained adequately to translate dietary recommendations into practical advice and to provide menu alternatives that consumers can understand and adopt. Students who plan to work in institutional food services must learn the techniques for adapting dietary recommendations to all aspects of food service management: menu planning, food purchasing, food preparation (including modification of recipes), meal service, and merchandising. Nutritionists and dietitians in food-service management positions have many opportunities to promote public health by helping both clients and food-service providers (e.g., cooks) fulfill their responsibilities to make more nutritionally desirable foods available to the public. As educators, nutrition specialists can help other health-care professionals acquire the information and skills needed to provide basic community nutrition education. Nutritionists and dietitians should be committed to following dietary recommendations and teaching others how to apply them wherever they work, including business and industry, private practice, academia, and government.

Physicians

A 1985 Food and Nutrition Board (FNB) committee concluded that nutrition education in U.S. medical schools is largely inadequate (NRC, 1985). Among the schools surveyed, it observed "a distinct lack of organizational structure and administrative support for nutrition programs" (p. 97). To ensure that nutrition programs become a permanent part of the medical school curriculum, the committee suggested that responsibility for them be vested in a separate department or division of clinical nutrition. The committee further recommended the establishment of a mechanism to monitor changes, if any, in the status of nutrition education in U.S. medical schools.

The 1985 FNB committee proposed explicit guidelines that would best incorporate principles of nutrition in the basic and clinical curricula of medical schools. Because the administrative structures of U.S. medical schools are so diverse, it was acknowledged that each school would be obliged to devise its own nutrition program, implementation strategy, and faculty structure. The committee recognized that a vigorous program in nutrition must always incorporate the latest investigative findings and that a mandated, inflexible curriculum is inherently outmoded. Nevertheless, it emphasized that certain broad areas pertaining to nutrition are an indispensable part of medical education. These areas include energy balance, the role of specific nutrients and dietary components, nutrition at different stages of the life cycle, assessment of nutritional status, protein-energy malnutrition, the role of nutrition in disease prevention and treatment, and any risks stemming from poor dietary practices because of individual, social, or cultural idiosyncracies (Weinsier et al., 1989). All these areas need to be rethought in relation to dietary recommendations, and the curriculum needs broadening to include elements of preventive medicine. For example, during the clinical training phase of medical school, students could learn basic nutrition counseling skills based on the communication/ persuasion and social learning models described in Chapter 3.

The number of U.S. medical schools with required nutrition courses dropped from 46 in 1981-1982 to 34 in 1987-1988 (Winick, 1989). Concomitantly, however, general nutrition education has been strengthened in most medical schools. The framework for an effective program is operating at the Emory University School of Medicine in Atlanta, Georgia, where an executive associate dean initiated a Nutrition Planning Committee composed of faculty from both basic and clinical science departments. All committee members have a professional interest in nutrition science, and all are active investigators in this field. The committee coordinates, advises, and participates in matters of curriculum design, recruitment of faculty in the area of nutrition, and guidance of the graduate degree programs in this field. It also supervises the coverage of nutrition throughout the campus. Furthermore, the committee coordinates its intramural activities with the other southeastern medical schools through SERMEN (Southeastern Region of Medical School Educators in Nutrition), which has a central office at the Medical College of Georgia in Augusta and a testing service based at the University of Alabama in Birmingham. Another apparently effective program is operating at the University of Texas Health Science Center in San Antonio (Young, 1988). A recent paper presents strategies to fit nutrition in the medical curriculum (Kushner et al., 1990).

Summaries and excerpts from the FNB reports *Recommended Dietary Allowances* (NRC, 1989b) and *Diet and Health: Implications for Reducing Chronic Disease Risk* (NRC, 1989a) as well as *The Surgeon General's Report on Nutrition and Health* (DHHS, 1988) should serve as resources for medical students learning about the relationships between nutrient intake and dietary patterns to the maintenance of health and risk of chronic disease. Other resources will be needed to teach basic nutrition concepts and such topics as nutritional therapies to treat specific diseases.

Nurses

At present, fundamental nutrition courses are not a prominent feature of baccalaureate or master's degree programs in nursing, although narrow elements of diet planning and disease-oriented diet therapy are incorporated into many required courses in the nursing curricula. Most programs that do provide nutrition courses are part of university medical centers such as the University of Washington (Seattle) School of Nursing (University of Washington, 1989). In the program descriptions of many nursing schools, there is no mention of nutrition education of patients as being a responsibility of nurses.

The inclusion of both basic and applied nutrition courses in nursing education has become increasingly important in light of the expanding roles of nurses in health care. Nurses often serve as the gatekeepers to patient care in primary health care units. In many clinical settings, for example, nurses conduct entry interviews, record pertinent historical details, act as triage coordinators, and frequently assume responsibility for the exit instructions regarding medications, diet, and other life-style changes. It is likely, then, that nurses (including registered nurses, nurse practitioners, and licensed midwives) working in various sites (e.g., hospitals, schools, clinics, and offices) can influence the eating habits of the public. To do so effectively, however, they must be adequately educated in nutrition, be sufficiently motivated to teach and encourage their patients to make dietary changes, and eat well themselves. Nurses have more daily contacts and interviews with patients in health-care settings than do those in any other professional group and thus have a great potential for influencing their clients.

Health Educators

Health educators work to promote health and prevent disease in state and local public service departments, even when their primary activities are geared to improving educational systems and social welfare or health-care policies. Their training should place additional emphasis on nutrition concepts and nutrition education methods to prepare them for their expanded roles in implementing dietary recommendations. Chairs of health education departments should draw on faculty outside the department with expertise in nutrition science and nutrition education to serve as instructors and advisers in the nutrition component of their programs. Practicing health educators should use the services and resources of food and nutrition specialists in their communities. In addition, they should improve their abilities to implement dietary recommendations by having access to electronic networks of nutrition literature and telephone or computer hotlines that could quickly provide them with accurate and practical information needed in specific situations.

More effective use should be made of another group of health educators—the more than 3,000 home economists with the Cooperative Extension Service (CES)—who disseminate nutrition information to consumers on an individual and group basis throughout the United States (Tope, 1990). In 1989, more than 10 million people participated in CES-organized nutrition programs, many of them provided through health departments, schools, churches, and local businesses.

Other Health-Care Professionals

Many other health-care professionals, including dentists, pharmacists, home economists, physician assistants, and medical epidemiologists, can be important sources of dietary information. All have unique opportunities to offer education and practical examples of the need for improved nutrition to their clients and colleagues. For example, dentists might inform their patients about diet-related measures for preventing and controlling dental caries, and pharmacists can help to disseminate the message that healthy people can and should obtain adequate amounts of essential nutrients by eating a variety of foods. Both can speak to colleagues and other health-care providers at continuing education programs about their successes and failures in promoting dietary recommendations.

STRATEGIES AND ACTIONS FOR HEALTH-CARE PROFESSIONALS

The committee developed three strategies and associated actions for health-care professionals to implement dietary recommendations.

STRATEGY 1: Raise the level of knowledge among all health-care professionals about food and nutrition and the relationships between diet and health.

ACTION 1: *Establish within the faculty of every health-care professional school an identifiable program with overall responsibility for planning and developing a research and education agenda in human nutrition.*

Considerable attention should be given to the nutrition education of physicians and nurses, since these two groups of professionals customarily represent the first contacts made by people seeking health care. These initial contacts, which number in the millions per day, are an excellent opportunity to provide patients with initial guidance and information about dietary recommendations. Patients who need more elaborate guidance or specific dietary modifications can be referred to qualified nutritionists and registered dietitians who have specialized knowledge and additional skills in this area.

One barrier to the successful implementation of this action is the limited number of faculty available to constitute an effective nutrition committee at most health-care professional schools. (Action 2 below is aimed at overcoming this barrier.) Another more difficult barrier is the institutional hesitation to expand curricular coverage (Nestle, 1988). However, an efficiently coordinated program might not require an increase in the hours spent on nutrition but, rather, an alteration of the existing hours by rearranging and coordinating coverage. A third barrier relates to coordination. In fields such as nutrition, which cut across many basic and clinical areas, some coordination with the curricula of related subject areas is essential but often difficult to achieve.

The establishment of an identifiable program with responsibility for planning, research, and education in human nutrition might be initiated by an individual school or be a cooperative effort among schools at a health center. A visibly supportive role by the university's administrative leadership is needed to ensure the success of the effort.

ACTION 2: *Establish a program within the Public Health Service to support the training of faculty in nutrition. The goal should be at least one nutrition faculty member per health-care professional school for each of the licensed graduate programs in the health-care professions.*

This program might be patterned after the current Preventive Cardiology Academic Award, which has been funded through the National Heart, Lung, and Blood Institute (NHLBI) at the National Institutes of Health (NIH) since 1979. It gives a competitively awarded 5-year grant to one faculty member in individual medical schools to develop programs in preventive cardiology. The grant provides up to 50% of the faculty person's salary plus funds to support the development and implementation of the program. The aim of the program is to have the school maintain the program after the completion of the 5-year period.

A nutrition award program could support a faculty member with clinical research interests in human nutrition. That faculty member would become an active member of the school's nutrition committee and would be expected to participate in all the campus activities related to nutrition. The award might be funded and administered by more than one NIH institute.

The major barrier, beyond the availability of funds, would be the maintenance of an active program on the campus after expiration of the grant. Limited availability of suitable faculty candidates for the award might also be a problem, but one that would diminish as more people in the various health-care professions devote themselves principally or exclusively to nutrition.

ACTION 3: *Materials emphasizing dietary recommendations for students in the health-care professions should be prepared by curriculum committees, authors, publishers, and others with interests in curriculum development. Such materials should include course syllabi at varying levels of complexity, batteries of examination*

questions, relevant bibliographic listings, audiovisual teaching instruments, and self-education computer programs.
Some clusters of schools (e.g., medical schools in the southeastern states) have already combined their resources in nutrition education and have made such teaching materials available to other schools (Feldman et al., 1989). A similar amalgamation of resources in clinical nutrition should be established for health-care professional schools.

Individual schools and faculty may wish to use only materials developed in house. Resistance to materials generated by outside authorities should be overcome, however, by the availability of authoritative reports such as *Diet and Health* (NRC, 1989a), *The Surgeon General's Report on Nutrition and Health* (DHHS, 1988), and the curricular materials developed by broad-based groups.

Clinical nutrition issues should be emphasized in such settings as informal nutrition rounds in both inpatient and outpatient settings, conferences, and formal seminars. Printed and audiovisual presentations should be made available to teaching institutions unable to develop such programs.

ACTION 4: *Expand nutrition education of health-care professionals at all levels. Certification and licensing bodies involved in the education of health-care professionals should require a demonstrated knowledge of nutrition.*
There is a need to increase the exposure of health-care professionals to clinical nutrition concepts in basic and graduate training as well as in continuing education. Students should be required to demonstrate their knowledge of nutrition and nutrition education methods by responding correctly to test questions on diet and health. Such questions should be incorporated into examinations assembled and sponsored by such professional bodies as the National Board of Medical Examiners (Winick, 1988). As a necessary step in bringing this about, professionals with expertise in nutrition should be asked to serve as advisory board members of licensing and accrediting agencies.

More continuing education programs in nutrition should be developed for health-care professionals. One useful example is *Rx Nutrition: Good Health in Practice*, a 2-year program designed to help physicians better understand connections between diet and disease and to provide them with practical guidelines to modify their own and their patients' eating habits (Health Learning Systems, Inc., 1989). This program is based on the recommendations in the *Diet and Health* report (NRC, 1989a).

Barriers to the acquisition of this new knowledge are both conceptual and practical, especially for physicians. Nutrition is not now identified as a specific component of most medical residency or graduate training programs (Boker et al., 1990). Certain medical specialties (e.g., gastroenterology and pediatrics) cover many elements of nutrition, but their coverage is rarely coordinated or focused. Another practical problem is that many programs in health-care educational institutions now compete for a limited allotment of teaching time. Furthermore, courses in nutrition do not yet teach students in most of the health-care professions the skills needed to motivate and enable people to make long-term improvements in their dietary patterns.

In medical schools, nutrition can be made part of the curricula in virtually all clinical areas (e.g., prenatal nutritional requirements in obstetrics). When nutrition is made an integral part of the broader program of preventive medicine, it is more likely to be accepted and maintained. Moreover, health-care practitioners should be encouraged to use the professional skills of registered dietitians and others with nutrition expertise in educating, motivating, and assessing the nutritional status of patients.

STRATEGY 2: Contribute to efforts that will lead to health-promoting dietary changes for health-care professionals, their clients, and the general population.

ACTION 1: *Encourage efforts to implement dietary recommendations in a coordinated manner for maximum effectiveness and to avoid unnecessary duplication.*

Two successful models have been developed for coordinating activities designed to control hypertension and hypercholesterolemia—the National High Blood Pressure Education Program (NHBPEP) (Roccella and Ward, 1984) and the National Cholesterol Education Program (NCEP) (Cleeman, 1989). Both programs were established under the direction of the NHLBI. Each consists of a coordinating committee composed of member organizations representing agencies within the federal government as well as major medical associations, voluntary health organizations, and various community programs. These committees mobilize and coordinate the resources and energies of participating organizations to achieve the goals of their respective programs.

The success of both NHBPEP and NCEP demonstrates that such coordination is feasible, enabling more effective overall attainment of goals, while avoiding wasteful duplication even as each member organization is encouraged to continue its individual efforts. A recent nutrition initiative based in part on the NHBPEP and NCEP models is Project LEAN (Low-Fat Eating for America Now). Sponsored by the Henry J. Kaiser Family Foundation (1988), its goals are to reduce the fat intake of the U.S. population to 30% of calories by 1998, to increase the availability and accessibility of low-fat foods, and to increase collaboration among national and community organizations in achieving these goals.

ACTION 2: *Encourage all health-care professionals to integrate nutrition information into their multiple counseling, treatment, skills training, and follow-up sessions with individual clients and patients.*

Health-care professionals should make the provision of nutrition information a prominent part of their hospital exit interviews and office visits with patients. In its recent report on health objectives for the nation, the U.S. Department of Health and Human Services (DHHS, 1990a) recommends that by the year 2000 at least 75% of primary care providers should routinely provide nutrition assessment and counseling to their patients or refer them to nutrition experts. Hospital rounds could also be used to educate both health-care professionals and patients about pertinent nutritional matters. Another means to implement this action is to establish standards for evaluation of nutritional status and instruction in clinical practice, particularly for such critical activities as pregnancy monitoring, child health visits, preemployment and school examinations, and clinical encounters with postoperative patients and elderly people.

It is important to note that this action cannot be implemented until third-party payers provide adequate reimbursement for nutrition counseling to compensate those whose skills and time would be required. Third-party payers must recognize the potential savings in medical-care expenditures that can accrue if nutrition information conveyed by health-care professionals reduces the prevalence of chronic disease in the United States.

ACTION 3: *Provide leadership, resources, and personnel for the dissemination of sound nutritional advice.*

Appropriate health-care professional societies should prepare and disseminate valid information to the media and serve as a permanent, readily available source for those seeking authoritative information and guidance on nutrition. In local communities, there are many opportunities for health-care professionals to carry out this function as individuals, through their professional societies, and through local affiliates of voluntary organizations. For example, they can take leadership roles in community organizing around nutrition issues; aid in the creation of a nutrition coalition or consortium that develops and coordinates local nutrition programs; and use newspapers, radio, and television to provide information and articulate their positions, thereby influencing consumer knowledge and behavior. (See Chapter 3 for a discussion of the media.)

ACTION 4: *Working as individuals or through professional societies, provide guidance to regulatory and legislative bodies concerned with the establishment of dietary standards and with rules and policies governing the production, harvesting, processing, preservation, distribution, and marketing of food products.*

Federal, state, and local legislators need to be better informed about nutrition and food issues. As members of national organizations and local communities, health-care professionals should offer guidance to policymakers on these subjects. For example, they might provide forums on food and nutrition issues for elected officials and link them with relevant activities or proposed initiatives in their local communities. The FNB, whose board and committees are composed primarily of health-care professionals, would continue to provide expert advice when called upon.

ACTION 5: *Specialists in human nutrition and food science, working through their professional organizations, should distribute practical information such as menus, recipes, and ideas for health promotion initiatives to private and public providers of meals.*

To implement this action, nutrition and food specialists should begin with their own hospital food services and branch out to school cafeterias, faculty clubs, commercial restaurants, nursing and convalescence homes, corporate dining rooms, and other appropriate settings. By providing this kind of practical information, health-care professionals may motivate meal providers to improve the variety of their menu offerings by including more nutritionally desirable foods and constructing meals that adhere to the principles of dietary recommendations.

ACTION 6: *Serve as role models by following dietary recommendations (and practicing other healthy behaviors) as often as possible.*

Health-care professionals should recognize that when they personally follow dietary recommendations, they are very likely to improve their own health and longevity, serve as role models for those who seek their professional guidance, and develop competence in the same self-management skills they must teach their patients. Therefore, the principles of dietary recommendations should be followed, for example, in the preparation of meals and snacks served at all meetings of health-care professionals, at client luncheons and dinners, at receptions, and in hospital cafeterias. One organization implementing this action is the American Public Health Association (APHA), which uses the *Dietary Guidelines for Americans* (USDA/DHHS, 1985) as a guide for planning meals and snacks at its meetings (APHA, 1987).

STRATEGY 3: Intensify research on the relationships between food, nutrition, and health and on the means to use this knowledge to promote the consumption of healthful diets.

ACTION 1: *Encourage sponsors of research to give high priority to research into diet and disease relationships and to developing innovative ways to use that knowledge in educating health-care professionals and the public about nutrition.*

In the public sector, intramural and extramural nutrition-oriented investigations should be stimulated through legislative, regulatory, and administrative channels. In the private sector, foundations, charities, and the food industry should be encouraged to participate in the underwriting of nutrition research. Unfortunately, although several public and private agencies and foundations fund nutrition research, few grants are primarily concerned with the dietary components of disease or in the educational and regulatory strategies to implement knowledge of diet and disease relationships.

Various food industry associations (e.g., the National Dairy Council, the American Meat Institute, and the Egg Nutrition Center) already fund nutrition research. There is a lack of industrywide collaboration in this direction, however, which may preclude the giving of needed attention to research areas that are not of interest to the individual grantors. Moreover, the credibility of research that is supported by industry groups may be questioned by many academicians and the public. Furthermore, the amount of money directed to research not oriented to specific products is very modest. Food and beverage companies are encouraged to collaborate to provide generous levels of untargeted funding. For example, if the food industry were to contribute substantially to a central, privately managed nutritional science fund, the research would be seen as more credible, and both industry and the public would benefit.

REFERENCES

ADA (American Dietetic Association). 1990. NCND thanks and welcomes corporate donors. ADA Courier 29(7):1.

Altman, L.K. November 28, 1989. How medical detectives identified the culprit behind a rare disorder. New York Times. C3.

APHA (American Public Health Association). 1987. APHA meal function guidelines for health conscious caterers. Photocopy. 1 p.

Boker, J.R., R.L. Weinsier, C.M. Brooks, and A.K. Olson. 1990. Components of effective clinical-nutrition training: a national survey of graduate medical education (residency) programs. Am. J. Clin. Nutr. 52:568-571.

182   *IMPROVING AMERICA'S DIET AND HEALTH*

CDC (Centers for Disease Control). 1989. Eosinophilia-myalgia syndrome—New Mexico. Morbid. Mortal. Weekly Rep. 38:765-767.
Cleeman, J.I. 1989. The National Cholesterol Education Program. Clin. Lab. Med. 9:7-15.
Council on Food and Nutrition. 1963. Nutrition teaching in medical schools. J. Am. Med. Assoc. 6:191-193.
DHHS (U.S. Department of Health and Human Services). 1988. The Surgeon General's Report on Nutrition and Health. DHHS (PHS) Publ. No. 88-50210. Public Health Service, U.S. Department of Health and Human Services. U.S. Government Printing Office, Washington, D.C. 727 pp.
DHHS (U.S. Department of Health and Human Services). 1990a. Healthy People 2000: National Health Promotion and Disease Prevention Objectives. Conference edition. Public Health Service, U.S. Department of Health and Human Services. U.S. Government Printing Office, Washington, D.C. 672 pp.
DHHS (U.S. Department of Health and Human Services). 1990b. Prevention '89/'90: Federal Programs and Progress. Public Health Service, U.S. Department of Health and Human Services. U.S. Government Printing Office, Washington, D.C. 192 pp.
Feldman, E.B., P.R. Borum, M. DiGirolamo, D.S. Feldman, J.M. Greene, S.B. Leonard, S.L. Morgan, J.F. Moinuddin, M.S. Read, and R.L. Weinsier. 1989. Creation of a regional medical-nutrition education network. Am. J. Clin. Nutr. 49:1-16.
Health Learning Systems, Inc. 1989. Rx Nutrition: Good Health in Practice. Sponsored by the University of Washington School of Medicine. Health Learning Systems, Inc., Little Falls, N.J.
Henry J. Kaiser Family Foundation. 1988. Project LEAN: Low-Fat Eating for America Now. Kaiser Family Foundation Health Promotion Program, Henry J. Kaiser Family Foundation, Menlo Park, Calif. 9 pp.
Kaufman, M. 1989. Nutrition services in state and local public health agencies, 1989: Preliminary report of biennial survey of state activities, 1989. Pp. 5-22 in Empowering Nutritionists for Leadership in Public Health. University of North Carolina, Chapel Hill, N.C.
Kushner, R.F., F.K. Thorp, J. Edwards, R.L. Weinsier, and C.M. Brooks. 1990. Implementing nutrition into the medical curriculum: a user's guide. Am. J. Clin. Nutr. 52:401-403.
Lenfant, C. 1986. A new challenge for America: the National Cholesterol Education Program. Circulation 73:855-856.
Nestle, M. 1988. Nutrition in medical education: new policies needed for the 1990s. J. Nutr. Educ. 20:S1-S6.
NRC (National Research Council). 1985. Nutrition Education in U.S. Medical Schools. Report of the Committee on Nutrition in Medical Education, Food and Nutrition Board, Commission on Life Sciences. National Academy Press, Washington, D.C. 141 pp.
NRC (National Research Council). 1989a. Diet and Health: Implications for Reducing Chronic Disease Risk. Report of the Committee on Diet and Health, Food and Nutrition Board, Commission on Life Sciences. National Academy Press, Washington, D.C. 749 pp.
NRC (National Research Council). 1989b. Recommended Dietary Allowances, 10th edition. Report of the Subcommittee on the Tenth Edition of the RDAs, Food and Nutrition Board, Commission on Life Sciences. National Academy Press, Washington, D.C. 284 pp.
Roccella, E.J., and G.W. Ward. 1984. The National High Blood Pressure Education Program: a description of its utility as a generic program model. Health Educ. Q. 11:225-242.

Tope, N.F. 1990. The role of Extension in helping Americans improve the nutritional quality of their diets. J. Food Qual. 13:55-58.

USDA/DHHS (U.S. Department of Agriculture/U.S. Department of Health and Human Services). 1985. Nutrition and Your Health: Dietary Guidelines for Americans, 2nd ed. Home and Garden Bulletin No. 228. U.S. Government Printing Office, Washington, D.C. 24 pp.

University of Washington. 1989. School of Nursing Undergraduate Curriculum Book. University of Washington, Seattle, Wash.

Weinsier, R.L., J.R. Boker, C.M. Brooks, R.F. Kushner, W.J. Visek, D.A. Mark, A. Lopez-S., M.S. Anderson, and K. Block. 1989. Priorities for nutrition content in a medical school curriculum: a national consensus of medical educators. Am. J. Clin. Nutr. 50:707-712.

Winick, M. 1988. The nutritionally illiterate physician. J. Nutr. Educ. 20:S12-S13.

Winick, M. 1989. Report on nutrition education in United States medical schools. Bull. N.Y. Acad. Med. 65:910-914.

Young, E.A. 1988. Nutrition education of medical students: problems and opportunities. J. Nutr. Educ. 20:S17-S19.

8

Education of the Public: Strategies and Actions for Implementation

S INCE EDUCATION about healthful dietary patterns can take place in so many settings and under so many different circumstances, the committee found it necessary to clearly identify the nature of the task to be undertaken before proposing recommendations for intervention. The recommendations developed in this chapter are directed toward individuals and families; home, child-care, and school meal providers; teachers and school administrators; educational and professional organizations; and federal, state, and local agencies or offices.

The analyses and recommendations in this chapter proceed from an understanding that education includes much more than schooling. This is neither a new insight nor a contested one. But left unstated, it is sometimes forgotten. Educators divide the broad term *education* into *formal, nonformal,* and *informal*— reflecting differences among the settings in which learning is assumed to occur. *Formal education* refers for the most part to schooling. The term *nonformal education* is usually applied to organized teaching and learning events that occur individually or in classes, for example, in community centers, in hospitals or clinics, and in maternal- and infant-care centers. *Informal education* refers to the almost infinite variety of educational experiences any society provides. Where food is concerned, these range from reading a newspaper article about dietary fat and fiber or watching food commercials on television to helping a parent cook dinner. The committee interpreted its mandate to include activities in all these educational settings, even though—as the above description indicates—this meant that the range of specific educational activities that could theoretically be considered was too large for detailed examination.

In light of the vastness of the domain to be surveyed, it was essential to specify the precise nature of the task to be undertaken. For this sector more than for any of the other societal sectors discussed in this report, the recommendations of the committee are constrained by the environment created by actions of the public and private sectors. The private sector and governments at various levels create and regulate both the actual foods available to consumers and most of the information about those foods that can be found in food stores, in fast-service and other eating establishments, and in advertising. This accounts for most of the information about food with which the average citizen comes into regular contact. Since consumers need to learn how to use available food and food information to enhance their health, much of the content of the lessons educators at all levels and in all settings must teach is delimited by an information environment created by the private and public sectors.

Some educators believe that education can affect both the availability of foods and the nature of the information available about them by altering consumer demand. To some extent, this is true. If educators had the resources to reach large groups of people, they could influence what such groups would or would not purchase. It is also unquestionably true that manufacturers cannot continue to produce a product that no one will buy—in that sense, consumer *demand* is essential. But manufacturers are also educators working, in Galbraith's term, to "manage demand" (Galbraith, 1967), and through their advertising they reach a much larger audience than that reached by professional educators. One consequence of this unequal contest is that consumer demand does not always lead manufacturers to produce the products or information actually needed.

A good example of this can be seen in the evolution of the market response to consumers' interest in the effects of diet on health. The particular safety and health concerns that emerged in the 1960s and 1970s were translated by some people into a desire to buy what they believed to be health-promoting foods, often at health food stores. The food industry responded to this interest by bringing into the market a succession of foods that were intended to be perceived as healthy—foods with designations such as *100% natural* or *organic*. Since neither the Food and Drug Administration (FDA) nor the Federal Trade Commission (FTC) had established regulatory definitions of the terms *natural* and *organic* (FTC, 1978), the consumer who attempted to identify health-promoting foods was confronted with food choices ranging from natural instant bouillon, natural yogurt chips, and natural batter-covered deep-fried onion rings to natural cigarettes (FTC, 1978; see also Belasco, 1989).

Consumers who later became convinced of the need to seek out or avoid certain specific components of foods could find products labeled and advertised as *lite, cholesterol-free, low salt,* or *high fiber*—designations that provided health guidance that was at best ambiguous and at worst misleading. So although consumers may be taught to demand certain kinds of foods and certain kinds of information about those foods, the marketplace may not respond in a manner really useful to those consumers, unless the regulatory apparatus helps it to do so.

Regulators who try to ensure that consumers are provided with clear information that enables them to make better food choices, thus making the food marketplace more *educationally transparent,* are constrained by limits on resources. Their task is also enormously complicated by the process of continual innovation that drives the market. Some sense of the difficulty of the regulatory task can be derived from a U.S. General Accounting Office (GAO) report entitled *Food Marketing: Frozen Pizza Cheese—Representative of Broader Food Labeling Issues* (GAO, 1988). This report sheds light on the complex relationship between the food supply, the food acquisition environment, and the role of the educator.

Frozen pizzas are regulated by both the U.S. Department of Agriculture (USDA) and the FDA—agencies that differ markedly in both their philosophies and their labeling requirements. The USDA (which regulates meat-topped frozen pizzas) has ruled that substitute ingredients need to be labeled as such only "if the analog ingredient changes the organoleptic characteristics [e.g., taste, odor, mouthfeel, color] of the product" (GAO, 1988, p. 30); i.e., only if the consumer detects a difference does the label need to reveal what causes it. The USDA guidelines thus permit a meat pizza to contain up to 90% cheese analog (usually made of casein, partially hydrogenated vegetable oil, salt, food starch, emulsifiers, stabilizers, and other additives) without triggering any special labeling.

On the other hand, FDA (which regulates frozen pizzas without meat topping) believes the public most needs information "where consumers cannot tell if the ingredient in question is 'real' or substitute" (GAO, 1988, p. 23). FDA, therefore, requires that a nonmeat pizza must contain *all* real cheese or indicate prominently on the label that it contains cheese analog.

Not only are the labeling requirements divergent, they are not even consistently enforced. When a GAO representative showed FDA a box of vegetarian pizza that contained cheese analog without being so labeled, the investigators were told by FDA that because of limited resources the agency could "focus only on labeling issues that can affect health and on the most flagrant and obvious labeling deceptions" (GAO, 1988, p. 30).

There is no agreement between the agencies involved or between their respective consumer advocates regarding the nutritional equivalence of real cheese and cheese analog. The example nevertheless dramatizes the consumer's dilemma. A consumer who believes that a particular cheese product is nutritionally superior and therefore wishes to select it may see side by side in the frozen food case two boxes: a cheese pizza prominently marked "Contains Cheese Analog," which might be composed of 90% real cheese, and next to it a meat-containing pizza or a vegetarian pizza that contained no such label—which could contain from 90 to 100% cheese analog. The consumer could easily purchase something she or he did not want.

The confusion of aims that this example suggests is, as the GAO report indicates, representative. Another example is the terms *lite* or *light*. FDA says that the nonmeat products it regulates must have 33% fewer calories than the regular version to be called *light*, while USDA says that the calorie levels need to be only 25% lower for the animal products it regulates (IOM, 1990). At the retail level, there is no consistent meaning for many food label descriptors such as *light*, *lite*, *lean*, *low fat*, *leaner*, and *lower fat*.

Despite this lack of uniformity and the confusion it produces, labeling has long been viewed by nutrition educators, consumer advocates, and sometimes by regulatory agencies as one of the most effective ways of helping consumers make informed choices. Because such a large proportion of the food supply is processed and packaged, there is no way for consumers to judge what they are buying except by reading what packages reveal about their own contents.

The preceding examples show that the agencies involved in regulating labeling do not at present agree even on the philosophy that ought to inform their regulatory thinking; e.g., should consumers be alerted when they are most or least likely to be misled by the organoleptic properties of a food product? If labels were more consistent, would consumers make more use of them? Which of the various pieces of information contained on food labels do they use and how well can they apply this information to such specific goals as reducing the fat content of their diets? These questions and others have recently been addressed to the extent possible (data are very limited) by another committee of the Food and Nutrition Board (IOM, 1990).

Information about specific food products can also be found in the mass media, largely in advertising. Television food advertising, especially that aimed at children, has intermittently aroused public concern and governmental attention since hunger advocate Robert Choate first testified in 1970 about the poor nutritional quality of breakfast cereals advertised to children (U.S. Congress, Senate, 1970). It has not been possible to devise a way to *prove* that food ads aimed at small children lead to poor eating habits, or that banning such ads would improve children's diets. Moreover, there is as yet no convincing evidence that public service advertisements or countercommercials for particularly nutritious foods can counteract the effects of advertising for less nutritious, so-called fun foods, at least partly because so few of these countercommercials have been aired (Smith et al., 1982). There is evidence, however, that antismoking countercommercials were successful enough to help drive cigarette advertising off the air (Erickson et al., 1990). The successful use of media as part of larger social marketing campaigns to encourage improved eating patterns is discussed in Chapter 3.

One official attempt to convert television food advertisements into carriers of nutritionally educational information was made in 1974 by the FTC in a proposed Trade Regulation Rule that would have required nutrition information in certain kinds of food ads (Tobin, 1974). Together with a companion initiative—a proposal to restrict some kinds of television advertising, including food advertising, aimed at children—the Trade Regulation Rule on Food Advertising provoked intense food industry opposition and subsequently a congressional refusal to approve the agency's operating budget. The regulation was ultimately abandoned (U.S. Congress, House, 1984).

Such regulatory efforts having failed, health-relevant information in food advertisements appears at the option of food manufacturers and their advertising agencies. As noted earlier, increased consumer interest in personal health has led to a considerable increase in health-oriented advertising. Currently, such advertising is constrained only by the requirement that it not purvey factually incorrect information, but even factually correct information may be misleading or difficult to interpret. For example, the claim that a vegetable oil-containing product is *cholesterol-free* does not help consumers learn that all vegetable oils derive their calories from fat, that only some of the fat is polyunsaturated, and that all are free of cholesterol. Almost inevitably, advertising offers "a truth" rather than "the whole truth" (Manoff, 1986), meaning—as the above examples illustrate—that even truthful information may mislead consumers by omitting other relevant information. While recently enacted food labeling legislation that gives FDA clear authority to regulate health claims on food labels does not directly apply to advertising (Food Chemical News, 1990a,b), it will undoubtedly influence how products carrying health claims on their labels will be promoted.

How can educators help consumers learn to make appropriate food choices in such a complicated and confusing information environment? Time-constrained consumers may not wish to master the rules for interpreting labels on the many thousands of processed foods in the marketplace, even if the labels were made more consistent and comprehensive. But perhaps consumers do not need to understand that many products. Each consumer, after all, buys only a minute portion of the 50,000 items (GAO, 1988) now on the market. Admittedly, consumers need to know only about the products they buy, but how are individuals who are to be taught about certain products to be identified? Individualized education is impractical. Thus, it is important to find rules of thumb that members of various sectors of the public can apply, without individual instruction, to any product they encounter in the marketplace.

As illustrated by the cheese analog, extra lean beef, and other labeling confusions, however, such rules of thumb are difficult to discover because decisions made by the private and public sectors have increased the complexity of the food supply and the food acquisition environment. In an environment glutted with small bits of data that do not readily coalesce into useful information, the only sorts of messages likely to be heard and remembered are simple, immediately useful ones. Yet how can simple truthful messages be devised that will enable consumers to make sense of a complex food supply?

As a mental experiment, we might imagine a world in which a single powerful individual could demand that nutritionists and consumer advocates create a system to place all foods into one of three categories: *Go*, *Caution*, and *Stop* (i.e., eat often; eat occasionally; and eat seldom, if at all). These foods would be marked with green, yellow, and red stickers. Consumers would be free to eat all red-labeled foods, but if they did so, they would at least be knowingly acting against the best advice of those trained to judge the nutritional worth of the food supply. Educating consumers to choose wisely in such a marketplace would be pleasantly simple, since it would be perceived that all the difficult decisions had been made by the nutritionists. (The decisions would have been difficult, of course, because nutritionists would have had much debate over which color of sticker to put on a food like potato chips.)

In June 1988, the American Heart Association (AHA) announced a plan to help consumers select foods as part of a balanced diet limited in fat, cholesterol, and salt (Graff, 1988). The plan proposed, which involved putting an AHA seal of approval on foods that met certain "heart-healthy" criteria, was in some respects similar to the imaginary marketplace envisioned above and it raised educationally relevant questions: Will consumers be misled into thinking that only AHA-approved foods are good and all others are bad? Will they think they can eat unlimited quantities of foods with an AHA seal? The program was never implemented, in part because of FDA and USDA objections that it would mislead consumers to think that labeled foods in a product category (such as fats and oils) were "good" and therefore could be consumed in unlimited quantities; similarly, unlabeled foods might be considered "bad" and thus avoided (Goldsmith, 1989). These objections illustrate some of the problems that an apparently simple solution to the consumer's dilemma can create.

Before considering other possible solutions to the need for simple messages in a complex marketplace, it is important to address at least one concern that the idea of very simple food labeling schemes might arouse in some readers—the issue of maintaining free choice. The necessity for free consumer choice is often emphasized by those who conceptualize education as a process of simply giving information. They argue that educators should not try to change behavior but, rather, should simply provide information that can be used by consumers in making their own food choices. As noted in Chapter 3, however, information alone is unlikely to be effective in changing dietary patterns.

Free choice is usually associated with the consumer's right to select from the largest variety of food products the market can supply. For example, the private sector has responded to the consumers' interest in health by adding new, healthier-seeming products to the market— not by withdrawing products that are attractive but less health-promoting. This presumably increases consumers' free choice.

In a democracy, however, free choice usually implies informed choice, and informedness and variety are to a large extent inversely related. The more products there are to choose from, the less time consumers have to learn about any one of them (e.g., choosing wisely from among 60 different yogurts is undeniably more difficult and time consuming than choosing wisely from among five different ones). Thus, the greater the number of choices, the more dependent the consumer becomes on either grasping at some single piece of information (e.g., avoid sugar, seek calcium) or trusting someone (e.g., the manufacturer, the advertiser, the newspaper food editor, the physician, the FDA, or the AHA) to provide a simple instruction to buy or reject a particular product.

In the imaginary marketplace described earlier, information available about products could include as many detailed facts, for example, about ingredients, nutrient composition, and manufacturing processes that any manufacturer wished to provide. The red, green, and yellow labels would simply signal to informed consumers that someone who cared about their health had judged this product a good or bad component of their diets. Thus, free choice would not be constrained.

Although most educators would probably be uncomfortable with a solution that asked so little of the consumer, knowledgeable teachers recognize that in *all* educational situations information is inevitably constrained. In educating about food, for example, it is not possible to give consumers information about approximately 50 nutrients (as well as the many nonnutritive substances that may affect their health) in each of the thousands of items in the food supply and to provide this information in a context that will enable individuals to relate their food choices to their health.

Yet a decision to give consumers some kinds of information and not others inevitably gives value to the information provided. Omission of information on the amount of added sugars or saturated fats in a product, for example, implies that these facts are less important in making food decisions than are the facts presented on the label (e.g., that the food contains no cholesterol). On the other hand, displaying the information that a given product contains 100% or some lesser percentage of the U.S. Recommended Daily Allowances (USRDA) for several nutrients may imply that nutrients not listed are less important or that the product so fortified is highly nutritious. All nutrition educators, whether they are professors or marketers, must always choose which information to include in teaching about diet and health.

Some selection of content must occur in all nutrition education, and in that selection process the educator inevitably expresses his or her assumptions—implicit or explicit—about which pieces of information will be important and useful to the learner. "Educating" is thus not possible if what is meant by that word is giving all the facts and nothing but the facts. Such dispassionate and unselective fact giving may appear theoretically desirable from the point of view of the discipline of education, but it simply does not exist in practice (Gussow and Contento, 1984, p. 18).

Consequently, the major unresolved question about how to teach consumers to implement dietary recommendations may not be whether consumer choice can be protected, since that is always limited in some way, but whether the particular simplifications required to teach this information can be made acceptable to all those who must cooperate in the enterprise. Objections to the imaginary marketplace, in other words, would not necessarily be based on a concern that such a signal system is too limited to give consumers real choice (since, as has been pointed out earlier, other information could still be available). Rather, such a system may be viewed as too simplified to be accurate, devoid of essential negative information, or practically and politically unattainable.

Nutrition educators might be happier with a less simplified marketplace in which the foods themselves were limited to commodities or simple recipe foods (e.g., bread) containing all or nearly all (and only) the nutrients such foods have traditionally contained. In such an environment, it would be possible to devise a simple food grouping method (with varying degrees of detail added for more educated consumers) for teaching food selection. Food education could be included in general education, beginning in the earliest grades with simple cooking and eating experiences designed to expand children's familiarity with, and liking for, different foods. An understanding of food composition and its relation to human health could be made part of the basic knowledge of all children and their parents and would be relatively easy to apply in the marketplace.

The six strategies and associated actions for implementation in this chapter must be read in light of these observations. Health-related information about relative or absolute quantities of specific food components should always be placed within an overall context that emphasizes food and food choices. It will continue to be difficult for the public to eat wisely when no simple and immediately self-evident rules of food composition are applicable. Success is most likely to be achieved if emphasis is given to the importance of choosing a diet from among health-promoting foods such as fruits, vegetables, grain products, lean meats, and low-fat dairy foods. It is much more difficult to teach consumers about products in which naturally occurring components have been concentrated or diluted so that the products can be labeled to appear more desirable. Most consumers are probably capable of learning to select and prepare foods wisely. The task, then, is to instruct and motivate them to do so.

STRATEGIES AND ACTIONS FOR EDUCATION OF THE PUBLIC

STRATEGY 1: Ensure that consistent educational messages about dietary recommendations reach the public.

ACTION 1: *Initiate meetings of leaders and representatives of national groups (e.g., interest groups, professional associations, and Cooperative Extension Service educators) to explore common interests in implementing dietary recommendations and to develop a series of common educational initiatives related to the attainment of that goal.*

Meetings of this kind, perhaps sponsored by a consortium of national health-related organizations, should decrease the tendency of opinion makers to focus on the differences rather than the similarities among various sets of dietary guidelines coming from such organizations as AHA and the American Cancer Society. Messages that reflect consensus will have greater impact and credibility, but each participating organization might be concerned that its identity would be obscured or its importance diminished in the eyes of its supporters if it joined this consortium. Since many of these organizations use interest in the disease that they were established to fight and publications addressing that disease to increase their own visibility and, hence, fund-raising ability, financial incentives may be required to foster cooperative efforts.

ACTION 2: *Review materials on diet and health prepared for the public by various professional groups and organizations to achieve consistency and ensure compatibility with dietary recommendations.*

The directors of professional groups and organizations should be prepared to approve the expenditures needed to revise their materials to emphasize dietary recommendations and how to meet them. This action is not intended to minimize individuality in style or emphasis on different diseases in redesigned educational messages. The need is for consistency in content only.

ACTION 3: *Convene an ad hoc committee composed of authors and publishers of leading nutrition textbooks to develop a series of broad guidelines that publishers could use to provide in their publications consistent and authoritative information on dietary recommendations and their scientific rationale.*

This committee would be convened to develop guidelines and materials on the connections between diet and health, on the food selection and preparation skills necessary to implement dietary recommendations, and on placing recommended dietary changes in the context of overall reduction of health risks. The products of this committee could be distributed to all major publishers in the fields of health and fitness, as well as publishers of the major texts in areas such as science, consumer education, home economics, social studies, psychology, and others that touch on nutrition or dietary patterns. These publishers would be encouraged to use the committee's guidance in developing new or revised publications.

ACTION 4: *Constitute a panel to review and evaluate nutrition education materials made available to schoolteachers from various food industry sources.*

In light of the chronic financial constraints that affect most schools, teachers are often tempted to use materials offered free or at low cost by various segments of the food industry—materials that may give incomplete or inaccurate messages and tend to promote brand-name food products, i.e., to "sell rather than teach" (Consumers Union Educational Services, 1990, p. 9; Harty, 1979). Teachers would benefit by having evaluations of such materials that come from a group of food, nutrition, and education professionals with access to a full range of relevant materials.

The materials should be evaluated to determine whether the content is explicitly and implicitly compatible with dietary recommendations. The results should be regularly updated and shared (perhaps on computerized data bases that are easily accessible) with state boards of education, with relevant educational associations, and with individual teachers considering use of particular materials. To improve the usefulness to schools of industry-produced educational materials, evaluations should also be sent on a regular basis to representative industry groups and various commodity, marketing, and trade associations.

There are no major barriers to this particular action item. A panel of reviewers may need minimal financial support, however, to cover travel, meeting, and other miscellaneous expenses. Other groups of professionals that evaluate various kinds of educational materials outside the food and nutrition areas may be able to provide guidance on establishing and maintaining such a review panel.

STRATEGY 2: Incorporate principles, concepts, and skills training that support dietary recommendations into all levels of schooling—kindergarten through college.

ACTION 1: *Design a model curriculum for teaching food skills, nutrition, and health from kindergarten through grade 12.*

Although a wide range of food, nutrition, and health education activities are currently undertaken in elementary, secondary, and high schools in the United States, they vary considerably in their level of educational sophistication. Overall, however, these activities tend to emphasize imparting *knowledge* of foods and nutrition rather than transmitting food coping skills, and they tend to focus—as has much of the dietary guidance to date—on basic commodities such as milk, meat, and produce. Thus, they do not adequately prepare children to deal with the extensively processed and packaged food supply of today. The proposed curriculum would attempt to overcome those limitations.

A food skills, nutrition, and health curriculum should be designed as a collaborative effort among such organizations as the Society for Nutrition Education, the American Dietetic Association, and the American Home Economics Association along with state departments of education and other relevant educational bodies of the various states. It should focus on (1) the role of a healthy diet in growth and development and in promoting vitality; (2) the ways in which foods are grown and processed and how these activities affect ultimate nutritional values through the loss or addition of nutrients or the addition of fat, salt, sugar, and water; (3) the development of skills needed to shop critically and to prepare quick, health-promoting meals or snacks from scratch; and (4) the importance of practicing other healthful behaviors (e.g., not smoking or using drugs and getting regular exercise) along with eating well. The curriculum should be designed as independent but interrelated modules so that separate topics could be taught if the entire curriculum could not be implemented.

In the early grades, such a curriculum might be designed to teach children the simplest concepts relating food intake to the growth and development of the body and acquaint them with various whole foods and simple ways of preparing them for consumption. In the upper primary grades, instructors could take advantage of children's innate curiosity about the world and themselves by teaching them in more detail about how their bodies use food to become and remain strong and healthy and teaching them about food production, processing, and marketing by providing food-growing experiences in classrooms or school gardens and by taking field trips to local farms, processing plants, and supermarkets. In the upper grades, lessons should emphasize providing adolescents of both sexes with personal survival skills that would help them achieve a high level of health and vitality through good nutrition. The goal would be to provide teenagers with shopping and cooking skills that would enable them to prepare and serve snacks and meals using whole grains, legumes, vegetables, and fruits.

The curriculum would be expected to provide a framework and examples of specific materials and methods that could be locally adapted and amplified. The extensive resources and holdings of the Food and Nutrition Information Center at USDA's National Agricultural Library will likely be of considerable help in developing the proposed curriculum.

Potential constraints to implementing this action include resistance to critical thinking about the ways food, nutrition, and health are currently taught; the difficulty of getting agreement among the educational organizations involved about the content and practicality of the curriculum; and resistance of some nutrition professionals to discussion of the negative aspects of some types of food processing.

ACTION 2: *During the development of the curriculum proposed in Strategy 2, Action 1 above, identify teacher-tested lessons— on health, nutrition, and food selection and preparation skills— suitable for use in a variety of classroom settings at different grade levels.*

This strategy would provide assistance to classroom teachers, who are most likely to teach subjects for which they have readily accessible age- and topic-appropriate lessons. Lessons could be coded to indicate where they fit at specific points in the curriculum and banked for eventual storage and retrieval on computer systems.

ACTION 3: *Professional nutrition, health promotion, and education organizations in each state should organize their members (and, through their members, local parents) to lobby state legislatures and urge state boards of education to mandate the inclusion of at least one food skills, nutrition, and health course in the requirements for teacher preparation in each state.*

Teachers inevitably tend to emphasize in classroom teaching those aspects of the curriculum with which they are most familiar and, hence, comfortable, and for which there seems the most urgent need. Since the food skills, nutrition, and health curriculum as envisioned would include units relevant to social studies, mathematics, science, home economics, and other topics, a teacher training course planned to illustrate the cross-disciplinary nature of the subject matter would encourage acceptance of the proposed curriculum—not as a new subject to teach but as an integrating focus in teacher preparation.

What might stand in the way? Nutrition tends to be regarded as part of health education. Hence, it competes for classroom time with topics such as sex, AIDS, drugs, and alcohol. There will be a tendency to continue to classify nutrition in this way and a consequent reluctance to add the new emphasis to an already crowded teacher training program. Therefore, implementation of this action may require the passage of legislation that will mandate its inclusion.

ACTION 4: *Revive, at the level of at least $0.50 per student, the USDA-administered Nutrition Education and Training (NET) Program that stimulated so much activity related to nutrition education in the late 1970s.*

The NET Program was created in 1978 to encourage good eating habits among schoolchildren and to teach them about relationships between diet and health (Kalina et al., 1989; USDA, 1986; see also Chapter 5). The program was originally funded at $26 million per year, or $0.50 per student. The NET Program overcame one of the major limitations to teaching nutrition in the classroom—namely, that most *functional* nutrition education (i.e., actual food selection) takes place elsewhere. The NET Program required a link between the classroom and the lunchroom. Funds were provided for training school food service personnel so that the children could try meals based on the lessons they had learned. Federal support for child nutrition programs, including the NET Program, was cut substantially in the early 1980s by laws designed to reduce domestic spending (U.S. Congress, House, 1988).

Congress, encouraged by lobbying by parents and professional associations, could revive the NET Program and provide it with adequate funding, even perhaps to the level of $1.00 per student per year, the funding level recently recommended by the American Dietetic Association (Hinton et al., 1990). The need for this action is great, because state and local school systems are unlikely to mandate or encourage the teaching of the proposed curriculum in the absence of resources commensurate with the task.

There are no substantial barriers to implementing this action, except continuing budget constraints, which may be a critical factor at a time of high deficits. However, since many schools have continued some pieces of initiatives begun under the NET Program, and much good curriculum material has been developed, even minimal funding would make it possible to increase the availability of these materials by bringing them into a clearinghouse. A new infusion of money into the NET Program would not be exhausted because of the need to organize a new system but would be used to restart a stalled one.

ACTION 5: *Offer a nutrition course or, at a minimum, a life science course with a well-developed nutrition component at institutions of higher learning.*

Many college students today desire accurate, meaningful information concerning nutrition and its relationship to health. In general, these are people who tend to be better read than others, and they frequently want useful, scientifically based information that is applicable to their daily lives. When a nutrition course is offered as part of a general education program, many students frequently elect to take it.

ACTION 6: *Offer each student in grades 7 through college on a periodic basis (e.g., every 3 years) a computer analysis of his or her diet and a professional evaluation of how the student's food habits conform to dietary recommendations.*

Traditional dietary analyses, which compare intake only with the Recommended Dietary Allowances (RDAs) (NRC, 1989), often fail to identify the major problems with young people's diets—excessive fat and salt intake and too few fruits, vegetables, and whole-grain products. By having their diets analyzed against dietary recommendations as well as the RDAs beginning in the higher grades, students can learn the importance of their food choices just when they are seriously beginning to manage their own diets. In addition, this procedure will enhance the personal relevance of diet and health messages and will thus encourage dietary change (see Chapter 3). If analyses are to be provided without cost to students through the food and health services of educational institutions, funds will be required to establish the programs, for staff training, for conducting the evaluations, and for providing student counseling.

STRATEGY 3: Ensure that children in child-care programs (including out-of-home care programs and family-, group-, or center-based programs) receive nutritious meals served in an environment that takes account of the importance of food in children's physical and emotional well-being.

ACTION 1: *Establish an interdisciplinary task force to oversee food-related matters involving children in child-care programs. This task force would include experts in pediatrics, nutrition, psychology, anthropology, and child development, along with child-care providers and parents.*
This task force could accomplish the following:

• Examine data on the diets and eating habits of preschool children of various economic, cultural, and ethnic groups and arrange for the collection of missing data in order to develop an overview of the present eating patterns of preschool children in the United States. Special attention should be paid to examining the effects of the changing compositions and life-styles of families on the diets and eating patterns of children.
• Assess the food programs of a sample of child-care programs from around the United States.
• Examine present standards for food and nutrition education training for health-care professionals, educators, and other people who provide care to preschool children, and determine minimally acceptable standards for such training.
• Explore ways of reaching new parents before their children are sent to child-care programs to emphasize the importance of providing children with healthful diets in wholesome settings. This can be accomplished by providing educational materials in maternity wards, in health-care settings, and at the workplace.

• Review the success and effectiveness of past efforts (e.g., the Head Start Program) and the current joint efforts of the American Public Health Association and the American Academy of Pediatrics in establishing nutrition standards for out-of-home care. Making use of lessons learned, develop national recommendations for legislation, regulations, and standards, as well as education and training guidelines for professionals and the public.

More than 56% of mothers with children under age 6 years and 61% of those with children ages 3 to 5 work outside the home (U.S. Department of Labor, 1989). An increasing number of these children are sent to child-care programs. There is only anecdotal information about the foods provided to these children by their parents for consumption during the day and few studies on what is served by child-care providers (Briley et al., 1989). There is even less information about whether or how these early food experiences help young children to develop a lifelong respect for both the physical and the emotional values of food. Health-promoting foods served in a nurturing environment are more likely to be accepted and enjoyed. Participatory education—that is, sharing good foods with caring adults in a pleasant environment—is the most powerful way of establishing healthful eating habits in preschool children (Birch, 1987; Birch and Marlin, 1982; Glaser, 1964).

Health-care professionals, early childhood specialists, policymakers, advocates for children, nutritionists, educators, and parents often lack awareness of how central food is to children's well-being. When the Child Care Development and Improvement bills (H.R. 3 and S. 5) were introduced in the 101st Congress, they carried no provisions for feeding children, training staff, or establishing nutrition standards for day-care settings. In at least one state there is a trend for child-care programs not to furnish food (Maryland Register, 1990). Ignoring preschoolers' food needs in child-care legislation will obviously save money if the bill becomes law, but it is clearly detrimental to the needs of children.

ACTION 2: *Public policy committees in nutrition, medical, and other health-related organizations should work to develop and pass legislation to require that foods served to children help them to meet dietary recommendations. The Child and Adult Care Food Program standard (USDA, 1990) should be used as a quality minimum.*

Members of the American Dietetic Association, the Society for Nutrition Education, the American Public Health Association, the American Institute of Nutrition, and the American Home Economics Association should work with members of the Alliance for Better Child Care to take the lead on this initiative. Given the budget implications of such a program, it will be critical to convince Congress of the importance of spending money early to help establish eating habits that may save money later through reduced health-care costs.

STRATEGY 4: Enhance consumers' knowledge and the skills they need to meet dietary recommendations through appropriate food selection and preparation.

ACTION 1: *Develop a consumer manual to present strategies that can be used to influence local food providers (and others who play important roles in the food system) to increase the availability of foods that help people meet dietary recommendations.*
The Society for Nutrition Education, the American Dietetic Association's National Center for Nutrition and Dietetics, the Consumer Federation of America, the Cooperative Extension Service, the Consumers Union, and perhaps other professional consumer organizations should be involved in preparing, publicizing, and distributing the manual. Such a manual would lay out general principles and strategies for:

• identifying reliable sources of information about food (e.g., the data bank discussed in Strategy 4, Action 2 below);
• making health-promoting food choices in, and influencing the menus of, local restaurants and other eating establishments;
• encouraging airlines and other travel-related industries to provide travelers with meals that follow the principles of dietary recommendations; and
• planning and implementing health-promoting eating events (both catered and noncatered), such as community potluck meals, fairs, festivals, and bake sales.

The consumer manual should also offer advice on how to influence other groups and individuals with the power to influence the food supply, for example:

• those in charge of selecting both the educational materials and the foods available in local schools, colleges, churches, health-care organizations, and hospitals;
• managers of local media who can be urged to present credible and useful information relevant to dietary recommendations (see also Strategy 6); and
• members of Congress or state representatives who can affect local or national food policies and regulations.

The public is bombarded by an enormous amount of information, much of which is of unknown reliability, and professional advice is not always readily available when decisions must be made. A manual such as that proposed would provide a reliable, self-explanatory (i.e., minimally mediated), and readily available source of needed information. The manual entitled *Reducing Dietary Fat* issued by Public Voice for Food and Health Policy (1989) is a useful, if restricted, model.

One possible barrier to the preparation of such a manual is the need to make it readable and usable by diverse populations with varying levels of literacy. This problem might be eliminated by preparing several versions of the manual that address different audiences. Publication and distribution costs might be underwritten by a publisher interested in selling such a volume at a profit.

ACTION 2: *Prepare an inexpensive, continually updatable foods data bank to inform consumers, food planners, and others about the nutritional content, composition, and production/processing history of the products available to them.*

Nutrition education professionals, food manufacturers, trade associations, food retailers, food technologists, consumer advocates, and appropriate government agencies should take the lead in establishing such a data bank as well as determining its content and format, relying heavily on the results of consumer surveys. Much of the needed nutritional information would be available from the USDA Nutrient Data Bank, an information system for storing and summarizing information on food composition (Perloff, 1989; Perloff et al., 1990). Additional information about the sources and processing history of a wide range of food products, including brand-name products, would need to be obtained from producers and processors.

The information should be presented in a format that facilitates comparison with a range of health-relevant criteria (e.g., content of saturated fat and cholesterol). The food and nutrition data bank could be made available in supermarkets, on floppy disks for use interchangeably in home or in store computers, or presented in such convenient forms as handbooks sufficiently inexpensive for consumers to purchase.

Although many consumers may not now be interested in detailed information about the composition, provenance, and processing history of their food products, the committee believes that the existence of a data bank containing such information and available in a variety of formats at different locations, including point-of-purchase settings, would fill a great need by generating consumer interest in the sources and compositions of foods. Studies should be initiated by FDA to determine which types of information in what kinds of formats could

202

IMPROVING AMERICA'S DIET AND HEALTH

be most readily used. Some formats for the presentation of food product information to consumers in magazine format are available, e.g., in the *Nutrition Action Healthletter* from the Center for Science in the Public Interest and *Consumer Reports* published by Consumers Union. Another example is the *Eat for Health Food Guide* issued by Giant Food, Inc. (1990), a Washington, D.C.-based food retailer.

Preparation of the data base may be impeded by incomplete information about various products and the difficulty of getting proprietary information from producers and processors. The rapid emergence and disappearance of products in the retail marketplace will make continual updating of this data base both a necessary and a formidable task.

STRATEGY 5: Establish systems for designing, implementing, and maintaining community-based interventions to improve dietary patterns.

ACTION 1: *Professional organizations concerned with food, nutrition, and health should work to engage community leaders in the development of community-based programs promoting dietary recommendations.*

Local affiliates of national professional organizations concerned with food, nutrition, and health should provide assistance to local schools, churches, work sites, hospitals, health departments, and community groups enabling them to (1) support on a local level the mass media and other national efforts to promote behavior consonant with dietary recommendations (see Strategy 6) and (2) revise their own organizational food practices to ensure that their offices and staffs serve as models of healthful dietary practices.

To achieve these goals, local community resources must be mobilized. For example, a key member of a local affiliate of the American Heart Association or the American Cancer Society can initiate the process of creating a coalition, consortium, or coordinating group to plan integrated community action in nutrition. Individuals from this group can then be appointed to serve as links to national resources. The most important barriers to such coordination arise from the territorial instincts of different community groups. Some fledgling community consortiums may require direct technical assistance to help them organize their communities to improve the nutritional savvy of their people. Assistance can be provided for organizing an assessment of community nutrition needs and an inventory of community nutrition resources, and for linking community groups as they become established to national and regional resources.

Once the organizational and planning barriers are overcome, the community nutrition consortium or coordinating council must deal with other barriers to implementation. One of these is the lack of trained personnel. Strategy 5, Action 2 below provides one logical means to remove this barrier.

ACTION 2: *Encourage schools of higher learning in various regions of the country to develop programs for educating and updating individuals in the skills needed to play key roles in community-based nutrition education programs.*
The training should focus on teaching methods of community organizing and program planning and on strategies for ensuring that community-based programs provide effective education. These programs should be rigorously evaluated for costs incurred and benefits provided.

Important components of the training programs should include how to (1) build coalitions gaining allegiance among all sectors of the community (i.e., interorganizational cooperation), (2) use and influence the media, (3) create incentive-based programs, (4) design point-of-purchase activities, (5) establish nutrition programs in schools and work sites, (6) develop methods for achieving regulatory and environmental change, and (7) ensure local relevance. Program faculty may need special training to enable them to design programs that meet the needs of their students and to evaluate their programs to ensure cost-effectiveness.

To properly evaluate the worth of community nutrition education programs, multiple methods will be needed. Low-cost telephone interviews could be conducted to evaluate consumer knowledge and determine self-reported behavior change. Measures that track the community's adoption (institutionalization) of program initiatives are needed, as are measures that track the secondary spread of influence (diffusion) of the initiatives. Local schools, work sites, hospitals, retail food suppliers, voluntary health agencies, health-care professionals, food producers, political bodies, and media organizations need to adopt new policies and methods to help members of the community maintain the improvements they make in their dietary practices that are likely to reduce their risks of disease. Lack of acceptance of this responsibility by local institutions and lack of resources for reinforcing the healthful dietary habits of community residents are indirect barriers to implementing this action.

STRATEGY 6: Enlist the mass media to help decrease consumer confusion and increase the knowledge and skills that will motivate and equip consumers to make health-promoting dietary choices.

ACTION 1: *Develop a series of social marketing campaigns to disseminate dietary recommendations.*

A model for such a campaign is Project LEAN (Low-Fat Eating for America Now), which is advancing the goal to reduce fat consumption. This project has been developed by Partners for Better Health with funds provided by the Henry J. Kaiser Family Foundation (1990) (see Chapter 7). Another model is California's "5 A Day—For Better Health" campaign, which is attempting to increase fruit and vegetable consumption among state residents to five servings per day and at least 500 lbs per year by the year 2000 (Foerster and Bal, 1990) (see Chapter 6). The promotion of specific dietary recommendations in social marketing campaigns should be placed within the context of overall risk reduction for chronic diseases.

The public and private sectors should collaborate whenever possible to support social marketing campaigns. The U.S. Department of Health and Human Services should examine sources of support for these campaigns that might include, on a national level, a voluntary $1.00 income tax checkoff, a stipulated percentage of food sales, a 0.5% tax on television food advertising, or a health lottery. At the state level, health promotion campaigns might be funded by so-called sin taxes on alcohol and cigarettes. California recently began a multimillion dollar campaign to reduce smoking in the state funded by a fraction of its cigarette tax revenues (Bal et al., 1990; Mydans, 1990). The results of this initiative should be monitored.

ACTION 2: *Appoint a committee of experts in nutrition education, child development, social influence, and media to review past attempts to regulate television food advertising to children.*

The committee's goal would be to recommend to Congress and the executive branch what, if any, action ought to be taken to ensure that the message stream reaching young children supports dietary recommendations. It might recommend (1) no action at all, (2) the introduction of messages to reinforce the food selection and preparation skills and nutrition lessons provided in the classroom, or (3) for very young children (ages 2 through 5), even a ban on the advertising of certain highly attractive foods whose consumption makes it difficult to meet dietary recommendations. Private foundations that might support the work of a children's television review panel could advocate that this action be implemented and provide some or all of the necessary resources.

In a recent promotion to food store managers, a well-known cereal manufacturer proclaimed that 95% of all children ages 2 through 11 would see a particular television spot promoting a particular cereal an average of 107 times within the first year of the cereal's introduction (Franz, 1986). Even allowing for advertising hyperbole, the campaign described is one of remarkable reach and frequency. Are the products being sold and the messages being delivered consonant with the principles of dietary recommendations for children? If not, does it matter? These are the sorts of questions the proposed panel would address. Although it is difficult to establish causal efficacy in regard to advertising aimed at children, it is nevertheless assumed to be effective by those who continue to advertise. The committee believes that growing congressional and parental concern over television advertising aimed at children and widespread awareness of nutritional problems such as obesity and high serum cholesterol levels among children make it vital to examine a variety of evidence and opinion on the question of whether these two phenomena are related.

Two barriers may impede this action. One is the conviction that nothing can be done to influence television advertising aimed at children, since past efforts have failed. The other is the pressure exerted by strong industry groups on Congress and the regulatory agencies.

ACTION 3: *Appoint a standing committee to coordinate the vast number of media activities necessary to increase consumer knowledge about dietary recommendations and their application and to decrease consumer confusion.*

Among the initiatives that this committee would undertake are the following:

• Arrange to produce an integrated set of public service announcements (PSAs) that carry simple, repetitive, and consistent messages designed to alert consumers to the health benefits of eating properly and the potential risks of not eating right and to direct them to reliable sources of information. Because PSAs are necessarily short and must compete for available air time with other good causes, they should attempt to convey awareness of issues rather than to communicate substantial nutrition information. Substantive information can better be conveyed through alternate routes once interest has been generated.

• Generate a list of media spokespeople, much like those who serve the Scientists Institute for Public Information, who will be available to reporters, feature writers, and editors to help them interpret the highly publicized reports about links between various isolated food components and disease that so confuse the public. These spokespeople should include people trained to clarify for food page editors how the new findings can be translated into food and cooking advice. The American Dietetic Association's Ambassadors Program and the Office of Scientific Public Affairs of the Institute of Food Technologists may serve such a role in certain contexts.

• Assist state dietetic associations to work with Cooperative Extension Service personnel to provide the national, regional, and local media—newspapers, weekly magazines, radio, television—with a weekly food tip, recipe, and menu designed to help people adopt dietary recommendations. Over radio and television, these tips could be provided by popular role models whose eating patterns meet dietary recommendations. Workshops should be conducted to train community leaders in techniques for working with their local radio and television stations and the local press to generate story ideas, assist with research, and provide resource people and materials.

• Cultivate contacts with the writers, directors, and producers of popular television series and movies, suggesting ways for them to plant messages (preferably implicit) about healthful diets within their programs. Bill Cosby, for example, idly munching a stalk of raw broccoli as he talks to one of his kids (or nuzzles his wife who is chewing an apple) would convey a much more powerful message than would any amount of explicit dietary advice. The promotion of less desirable behavior was used successfully in the 1950s by modeling to glamorize smoking (Erickson et al., 1990) and more recently to promote brand-name products such as soft drinks and beer (Miller, 1990). Recently, the tobacco industry has paid movie producers to portray smokers in movies and to film particular brands of cigarettes (Miller, 1990). The placement of brand-name products in movies and television programs is a large and growing business (Miller, 1990). Yet there is little or no modeling of appropriate dietary behavior in television shows heavily watched by young people. One recent survey of 11 top-ranked prime-time television series found "pervasive" references to food in the programs and the accompanying commercials; in most cases, the foods shown were of low nutritional quality and consumed between meals (Story and Faulkner, 1990). Success in obtaining the cooperation of producers to discourage driving after drinking alcoholic beverages on popular television shows has been achieved by Dr. Jay A. Winsten and his colleagues from the Harvard Center for Health Communication (DeJong and Winsten, 1990).

• Retain a skilled public relations consultant to place guests, anecdotes, and stories on radio and television talk shows, news and news magazine shows, and game shows in support of healthful dietary patterns. Such placements should be carefully planned so that the diet and health messages are supported both explicitly and implicitly by the appearance and reputation of the spokespeople.

Although paid advertising, especially on television, has been used successfully to sell food products, there have been few efforts to date to use the national and local mass media in an organized way to promote healthful eating. Since a large portion of the information on all subjects that reaches the U.S. public comes explicitly or implicitly through the media, the need to engage this sector in promoting healthful eating behaviors is evident.

Two major barriers to implementing this action are the large cost of an initiative of the size described and the resistance of large and powerful segments of the food industry to negative statements about its food or beverage products.

ACTION 4: *Establish a task force of social scientists to examine the utility of national entertainment television as a community-organizing tool that can be used to enhance efforts of local health agencies in encouraging appropriate dietary changes.*

Television tends to be viewed primarily as entertainment and very secondarily as an educational medium. The only sustained attempt in the United States to use national television to modify eating behavior in a healthful direction (among other goals) was "Feeling Good," a Children's Television Workshop health show that aired in 1974 and 1975. Although the show was critically judged to be a failure, it apparently provided community organizations with an opportunity to organize around specific health issues. There is evidence that several of its nutrition messages were effective (Levine and Gussow, in press), even though the intended programming was never completed.

REFERENCES

Bal, D.G., K.W. Kizer, P.G. Felten, H.N. Mozar, and D. Niemeyer. 1990. Reducing tobacco consumption in California: development of a statewide anti-tobacco use campaign. J. Am. Med. Assoc. 264:1570-1574.

Belasco, W.J. 1989. Appetite for Change: How the Counterculture Took on the Food Industry, 1966-1988. Pantheon Books, New York. 311 pp.

Birch, L.L. 1987. The role of experience in children's food acceptance patterns. J. Am. Diet. Assoc. 87:S36-S40.

Birch, L.L., and D.W. Marlin. 1982. I don't like it; I never tried it: effects of exposure on two-year-old children's food preferences. Appetite 3:353-360.

Briley, M.E., A.C. Buller, C. R. Roberts-Gray, and A. Sparkman. 1989. What is on the menu at the child care center? J. Am. Diet. Assoc. 89:771-774.

Consumers Union Educational Services. 1990. Selling America's Kids: Commercial Pressures on Kids in the 90's. Consumers Union of United States, Inc., Mount Vernon, N.Y. 23 pp.

DeJong, W., and J.A. Winsten. 1990. The use of mass media in substance abuse prevention. Health Affairs 9:30-46.

Erickson, A.C., J.W. McKenna, and R.M. Romano. 1990. Past lessons and new uses of the mass media in reducing tobacco consumption. Public Health Rep. 105:239-244.

Foerster, S.B., and D.G. Bal. 1990. California's "5 A Day—For Better Health" campaign. Chronic Dis. Notes Rep. 3(1):7-9.

Food Chemical News. 1990a. Health claims additional re-proposal seen likely. Food Chem. News 32(37):3-6.

Food Chemical News. 1990b. Hutt hits need for FDA clearance of new health messages. Food Chem. News 32(37):43-45.

FTC (Federal Trade Commission). 1978. Proposed Trade Regulation Rule on Food Advertising. Phase I. Staff Report and Recommendations. Federal Trade Commission, Washington, D.C. 367 pp.

Franz, J. 1986. General Mills pours out 3rd cereal. Advertising Age 57:2.

GAO (U.S. General Accounting Office). 1988. Food Marketing: Frozen Pizza Cheese— Representative of Broader Food Labeling Issues. Report No. GAO/RCED-88-70. U.S. General Accounting Office, Washington, D.C. 47 pp.

Galbraith, J.K. 1967. The New Industrial State. Houghton Mifflin, Boston. 427 pp.

Giant Food, Inc. 1990. Eat for Health Food Guide. Giant Food, Inc., Landover, Md. 230 pp.

Glaser, A. 1964. Nursery school can influence foods acceptance. J. Home Econ. 56:680-683.

Goldsmith, M.F. 1989. 'HeartGuide' food-rating program attracts 114 applications as controversy continues. J. Am. Med. Assoc. 262:3388, 3391.

Graff, V. 1988. "A bold move": AHA to begin approving food products in 1989. Am. Heart News 5:2-4, 11.

Gussow, J.D., and I. Contento. 1984. Nutrition education in a changing world. World Rev. Nutr. Diet. 44:1-56.

Harty, S. 1979. Hucksters in the Classroom: A Review of Industry Propaganda in Schools. Center for Study of Responsive Law, Washington, D.C. 190 pp.

Henry J. Kaiser Family Foundation. 1990. Idea Kit for State and Community Programs to Reduce Dietary Fat. Project LEAN: Low-Fat Eating for America Now. Henry J. Kaiser Family Foundation, Menlo Park, Calif. 126 pp.

Hinton, A.W., J. Heimindinger, and S.B. Foerster. 1990. Position of the American Dietetic Association: domestic hunger and inadequate access to food. J. Am. Diet. Assoc. 90:1437-1441.

IOM (Institute of Medicine). 1990. Nutrition Labeling: Issues and Directions for the 1990s. Report of the Committee on Nutrition Components of Food Labeling, Food and Nutrition Board. National Academy Press, Washington, D.C. 355 pp.

Kalina, B.B., C.A. Philipps, and H.V. Minns. 1989. The NET Program: a ten-year perspective. J. Nutr. Educ. 21:38-42.

Levine, J., and J.D. Gussow. In press. Better than we think? A reassessment of "Feeling Good." J. Nutr. Educ.

Manoff, R.K. 1986. Health claim? Less is best. Advertising Age 57:18, 22.

Maryland Register. 1990. Child Care Center Licensing. Title 07, Office of Child Care Licensing and Regulation, Department of Human Resources. Md. Reg. 17:1362-1374.

Miller, M.C. 1990. Advertising: end of story. Pp. 186-246 in M.C. Miller, ed. Seeing Through Movies. Pantheon Books, New York.

Mydans, S. April 11, 1990. California uses tobacco tax for ads attacking smoking. New York Times. A1, B5.

NRC (National Research Council). 1989. Recommended Dietary Allowances, 10th edition. Report of the Subcommittee on the Tenth Edition of the RDAs, Food and Nutrition Board, Commission on Life Sciences. National Academy Press, Washington, D.C. 284 pp.

Perloff, B.P. 1989. Analysis of dietary data. Am. J. Clin. Nutr. 50:1128-1132.

Perloff, B.P., R.L. Rizek, D.B. Haytowitz, and P.R. Reid. 1990. Dietary intake methodology II. USDA's Nutrient Data Base for Nationwide Dietary Intake Surveys. J. Nutr. 120:1530-1534.

Public Voice for Food and Health Policy. 1989. Reducing Dietary Fat: Strategies for State and Local Community Leaders. Public Voice for Food and Health Policy, Washington, D.C. 14 pp.

Smith, K.W., S.K. Nelson, and J.J. O'Hara. 1982. Food for Thought Project: Final Report. Office of Policy, Planning and Evaluation, Food and Nutrition Service, U.S. Department of Agriculture, Alexandria, Va. 95 pp.

Story, M., and P. Faulkner. 1990. The prime time diet: a content analysis of eating behavior and food messages in television program content and commercials. Am. J. Public Health 80:738-740.

Tobin, C.A. 1974. Food advertising: proposed trade regulation rule. Fed. Reg. 39:39842-39862.

U.S. Congress, House. 1984. FTC Review (1977-84). Subcommittee on Oversight and Investigations, Committee on Energy and Commerce, Subcommittee on Oversight and Investigations, U.S. House of Representatives. Committee Print 98-CC. U.S. Government Printing Office, Washington, D.C. 394 pp.

U.S. Congress, House. 1988. Child Nutrition Programs: Issues for the 101st Congress. Subcommittee on Elementary, Secondary, and Vocational Education, Committee on Education and Labor, U.S. House of Representatives. Serial No. 100-CC. U.S. Government Printing Office, Washington, D.C. 220 pp.

U.S. Congress, Senate. 1970. Open Hearing re. Nutritional Aspects of Dry Breakfast Cereals and the Related Advertising Practices of Cereal Manufacturers. Subcommittee on the Consumer, Committee on Commerce, U.S. Senate. Hearing No. 91-72. U.S. Government Printing Office, Washington, D.C. 284 pp.

USDA (U.S. Department of Agriculture). 1986. USDA Comprehensive Plan for a National Food and Human Nutrition Research and Education Program. A Report to Congress. Publication 1987-180-917/60064. U.S. Government Printing Office, Washington, D.C. 91 pp.

USDA (U.S. Department of Agriculture). 1990. Child and Adult Care Food Program. U.S. Department of Agriculture, Alexandria, Va. 5 pp.

U.S. Department of Labor. 1989. Handbook of Labor Statistics. Bulletin 2340, August 1989. U.S. Bureau of Labor Statistics, Washington, D.C.

9

Directions for Research

A S INDICATED throughout this report, continued research is essential to establish a better base of knowledge for designing effective and efficient implementation strategies and for assessing their costs and benefits. The committee identified six principal areas of research in which more activity is required to achieve these goals. They are not ranked in any order of priority. In the committee's judgment, successful implementation requires that research in all six areas be conducted simultaneously, as is currently the case. In fact, there is considerable overlap between the research areas because each is broad in scope and complex to investigate.

Research in each of the areas identified below tends to be conducted by different types of experts in a wide variety of settings, including nutrition scientists in laboratories; public health specialists in communities; food policy analysts working for governments, voluntary agencies, and consumer advocacy groups; and economists and other social scientists in schools of higher education. Resources to increase research in these areas will need to come from a wide variety of sources, including governments, the private sector, foundations, voluntary agencies, and academia.

1. Improve methods to characterize what people actually eat, especially over long periods during which dietary patterns change.

The difficulty in assessing dietary intakes is a major impediment in studying the effects of diet on health and on assessing the effects of initiatives to improve eating habits. There are weaknesses in all current assessment methods (e.g., those based on food disappearance, household food inventories, and individual diet histories) (see review in the *Diet and Health* report [NRC, 1989, Chapter 2]). More comprehensive data collection and timely reporting of results are required to learn more about what people eat and how eating habits vary in relation to such factors as geographical location, life-style, ethnicity, and socioeconomic status. High priority should be given to improving methods for collecting and assessing data on dietary patterns, including the intakes of specific foods and the dietary constituents of foods (e.g., macro- and microconstituents that affect the risk of chronic diseases).

2. Increase understanding of the existing and potential determinants of dietary change and how this knowledge can be used to promote more healthful eating behaviors.

As noted in Chapter 3, much more needs to be learned about the behaviors and motivations of people who have improved their diets compared with the behaviors and motivations of those who have not and how dietary change is most effectively induced. Research in this area would include basic and applied studies to lead to better understanding of the obstacles to, and opportunities for, dietary change. In addition, very little is known about the influence of major life-style factors (e.g., moving out of the parents' home, getting married, having children, and working in a demanding job) on dietary changes. Studies should also be conducted to learn more about taste preferences and how dietary change is influenced by the media (especially television), growing older, and genetic and cultural factors. Furthermore, the extent to which environmental factors affect dietary change require investigation. These factors include proximity of grocery stores of various sizes to shoppers, transportation facilities, food costs, low-income-neighborhood shopping strategies, and security of shopping areas. Learning more about why, how, and when during the course of a lifetime people began to adopt more healthful diets would provide a better understanding of the factors that lead to long-term dietary change (Achterberg and Trenkner, 1990; Sims, 1987; Sims and Light, 1980).

Major efforts have been undertaken to educate and motivate people to practice healthy behaviors such as quitting smoking or refraining from taking up the habit, fastening seat belts in the car, and not driving after drinking alcoholic beverages. Research should be conducted to determine how the lessons learned from these initiatives can be applied to the task of improving U.S. dietary patterns.

3. Continue research to develop new food products and modify both the production and processing of existing products to help consumers more easily meet dietary recommendations.

By applying the results of research conducted at government, industry, and academic facilities, various segments of the food industry have been able to develop nutritionally desirable foods that help consumers to more easily meet dietary recommendations (see Chapter 6). This research should continue, especially in the areas of flavor, texture, nutrient content and retention, preservation, and safety. Perhaps the food industry could respond to trends (or anticipate them) even more readily if more research were conducted to track consumer attitudes and knowledge about food and nutrition issues and about their food selection and preparation practices. Research should also be conducted to identify alternative uses of foods or food constituents (e.g., butterfat) that should be limited in a healthful diet.

4. Review and improve government and private-sector policies that directly and indirectly affect the availability of particular foods and the promotion of healthful dietary patterns.

As noted throughout this report, government policies and private-sector practices substantially influence consumer food demands and dietary patterns—often in complex and subtle ways. Systematic and comprehensive studies should be conducted to determine precisely how and at what critical points the policies and practices are so influential. Studies should include comprehensive reviews of public laws and regulations and private-sector activities pertaining to food and nutrition. For example, there is a need to reconcile government activities in these areas at the federal, state, and local levels. Results could be used to improve policies and practices so that they encourage acceptance and practice of dietary recommendations.

5. Determine how implementors of dietary recommendations at all levels (e.g., supermarket managers, physicians, and high school health teachers) can more effectively teach the basis of the recommendations and motivate people to follow them.

Success in implementing dietary recommendations can be achieved only by teaching their basis and application to people with different levels of interest in improving their diets, different capacities for understanding the recommendations themselves, and different tendencies to become either informed, confused, or overwhelmed by the proliferation of information and promotions encouraging consumption of particular food products. Continued research is required to develop educational strategies that motivate and empower people to select and consume healthful diets that are nutritionally adequate and meet dietary recommendations.

6. Investigate the costs and benefits of implementing dietary recommendations as proposed by this committee and by others.

As described in Chapter 2, scarce financial and human resources should be used efficiently to accomplish the goals of implementation at the lowest costs. The committee discovered that it could not provide estimates of the costs and benefits of its recommendations primarily because of the lack of quantification of the effects of past initiatives to improve dietary practices. In order to make cost-benefit calculations, the following types of systematic documentation are needed: (1) the amount, length, and frequency of exposure to food and nutrition messages; (2) descriptions of the channels through which the messages are provided; and (3) the effects of the messages in terms of knowledge, attitude, and behavioral changes of recipients. Continued research to determine effective and efficient means to evaluate initiatives to implement dietary recommendations is important. In addition, all initiatives to improve dietary patterns should include a comprehensive evaluation component and sufficient resources to carry it out; the descriptions and results of these evaluations should be made publicly available.

REFERENCES

Achterberg, C., and L.L. Trenkner. 1990. Developing a working philosophy of nutrition education. J. Nutr. Educ. 22:189-193.

NRC (National Research Council). 1989. Diet and Health: Implications for Reducing Chronic Disease Risk. Report of the Committee on Diet and Health, Food and Nutrition Board, Commission on Life Sciences. National Academy Press, Washington, D.C. 749 pp.

Sims, L.S. 1987. Nutrition education research: reaching toward the leading edge. J. Am. Diet. Assoc. 87:S10-S18.

Sims, L.S., and L. Light. 1980. Directions for Nutrition Education Research: The Penn State Conferences: A Proceeding. Pennsylvania State University, University Park, Pa. 108 pp.

A

Dietary Recommendations

As described in Chapters 1 and 2, the term *dietary recommendations* is used throughout this report to refer as a group to the dietary advice in (1) the *Diet and Health* report of the Food and Nutrition Board of the National Academy of Sciences, (2) *The Surgeon General's Report on Nutrition and Health,* and (3) the *Dietary Guidelines for Americans* report by the U.S. Departments of Agriculture and Health and Human Services. These three sets of dietary guidance are presented below.

RECOMMENDATIONS FROM THE *DIET AND HEALTH* REPORT[1]

1. Reduce total fat intake to 30% or less of calories. Reduce saturated fatty acid intake to less than 10% of calories, and the intake of cholesterol to less than 300 mg daily. The intake of fat and cholesterol can be reduced by substituting fish, poultry without skin, lean meats, and low- or nonfat dairy products for fatty meats and whole-milk dairy products; by choosing more vegetables, fruits, cereals, and legumes; and by limiting oils, fats, egg yolks, and fried and other fatty foods.

2. Every day eat five or more servings of a combination of vegetables and fruits, especially green and yellow vegetables and citrus fruits. Also, increase intake of starches and other complex carbohydrates by eating six or more daily servings of a combination of breads, cereals, and legumes.

3. Maintain protein intake at moderate levels.

4. Balance food intake and physical activity to maintain appropriate body weight.

5. The committee does not recommend alcohol consumption. For those who drink alcoholic beverages, the committee recommends limiting consumption to the equivalent of less than 1 ounce of pure alcohol in a single day. This is the equivalent of two cans of beer, two small glasses of wine, or two average cocktails. Pregnant women should avoid alcoholic beverages.

6. Limit total daily intake of salt (sodium chloride) to 6 g or less. Limit the use of salt in cooking and avoid adding it to food at the table. Salty, highly processed salty, salt-preserved, and salt-pickled foods should be consumed sparingly.

7. Maintain adequate calcium intake.

8. Avoid taking dietary supplements in excess of the RDA [Recommended Dietary Allowances[2]] in any one day.

9. Maintain an optimal intake of fluoride, particularly during the years of primary and secondary tooth formation and growth.

RECOMMENDATIONS OF THE SURGEON GENERAL OF THE UNITED STATES[3]

Issues for Most People

1. *Fats and cholesterol:* Reduce consumption of fat (especially saturated fat) and cholesterol. Choose foods relatively low in these substances, such as vegetables, fruits, whole grain foods, fish, poultry, lean meats, and low-fat dairy products. Use food preparation methods that add little or no fat.

2. *Energy and weight control:* Achieve and maintain a desirable body weight. To do so, choose a dietary pattern in which energy (caloric) intake is consistent with energy expenditure. To reduce energy intake, limit consumption of foods relatively high in calories, fats, and sugars, and minimize alcohol consumption. Increase energy expenditure through regular and sustained physical activity.

3. *Complex carbohydrates and fiber:* Increase consumption of whole grain foods and cereal products, vegetables (including dried beans and peas), and fruits.

4. *Sodium:* Reduce intake of sodium by choosing foods relatively low in sodium and limiting the amount of salt added in food preparation and at the table.

5. *Alcohol:* To reduce the risk for chronic disease, take alcohol only in moderation (no more than two drinks a day), if at all. Avoid

drinking any alcohol before or while driving, operating machinery, taking medications, or engaging in any other activity requiring judgment. Avoid drinking alcohol while pregnant.

Other Issues for Some People

6. *Fluoride:* Community water systems should contain fluoride at optimal levels for prevention of tooth decay. If such water is not available, use other appropriate sources of fluoride.

7. *Sugars:* Those who are particularly vulnerable to dental caries (cavities), especially children, should limit their consumption and frequency of use of foods high in sugars.

8. *Calcium:* Adolescent girls and adult women should increase consumption of foods high in calcium, including low-fat dairy products.

9. *Iron:* Children, adolescents, and women of childbearing age should be sure to consume foods that are good sources of iron, such as lean meats, fish, certain beans, and iron-enriched cereals and whole grain products. This issue is of special concern for low-income families.

DIETARY GUIDELINES FOR AMERICANS[4]

1. Eat a variety of foods.
2. Maintain healthy weight.
3. Choose a diet low in fat, saturated fat, and cholesterol.
4. Choose a diet with plenty of vegetables, fruits, and grain products.
5. Use sugars only in moderation.
6. Use salt and sodium only in moderation.
7. If you drink alcoholic beverages, do so in moderation.

NOTES

1. Source: National Research Council. 1989. Diet and Health: Implications for Reducing Chronic Disease Risk. Report of the Committee on Diet and Health, Food and Nutrition Board, Commission on Life Sciences. National Academy Press, Washington, D.C. 749 pp.

2. National Research Council. 1989. Recommended Dietary Allowances, 10th ed. Report of the Subcommittee on the Tenth Edition of the RDAs, Food and Nutrition Board, Commission on Life Sciences. National Academy Press, Washington, D.C. 284 pp.

3. Source: U.S. Department of Health and Human Services. 1988. The Surgeon General's Report on Nutrition and Health. DHHS (PHS) Publ. No. 88-50210. Public Health Service, U.S. Department of Health and Human Services. U.S. Government Printing Office, Washington, D.C. 727 pp.

4. Source: U.S. Department of Agriculture/U.S. Department of Health and Human Services. 1990. Nutrition and Your Health: Dietary Guidelines for Americans, 3rd ed. Home & Garden Bulletin No. 232. U.S. Department of Agriculture and U.S. Department of Health and Human Services, Washington, D.C. 28 pp.

APPENDIX

B

Summary of Committee's Major Recommendations

PRINCIPAL IMPLEMENTATION STRATEGIES

1. Governments and health-care professionals must become more active as policymakers, role models, and agenda setters in implementing dietary recommendations.
2. Improve the nutrition knowledge of the public and increase the opportunities to practice good nutrition.
3. Increase the availability of health-promoting food.

RECOMMENDATIONS TO THE PUBLIC SECTOR

STRATEGY 1: Improve federal efforts to implement dietary recommendations.

ACTION 1: *The executive branch should establish a coordinating mechanism that would promote the implementation of dietary recommendations.*

ACTION 2: *Encourage members of the U.S. Congress and state legislative bodies to play active roles in the implementation of dietary recommendations.*

STRATEGY 2: Alter federal programs that directly influence what Americans eat so as to encourage rather than impede the implementation of dietary recommendations. This effort should affect food assistance, food safety, and

nutrition programs, as well as farm subsidy, tariff, and trade programs.

ACTION 1: *Revise current U.S. Department of Agriculture (USDA) regulations governing the child and family nutrition programs to comply with dietary recommendations and train federal, regional, state, and local personnel administering the programs to implement the recommendations.*

ACTION 2: *Revise current regulations governing the Nutrition Program for Older Americans (which provides congregate meals and home-delivered meals) to conform to the principles of dietary recommendations and train federal, regional, state, and local personnel administering the programs accordingly.*

ACTION 3: *USDA and the U.S. Department of Health and Human Services (DHHS) should ensure that food and health programs serving all special populations conform to dietary recommendations.*

ACTION 4: *Ensure that the education and information components of the foregoing federal food assistance and nutrition programs are consistent with dietary recommendations.*

ACTION 5: *Incorporate dietary recommendations into current rules and regulations governing commodity purchases.*

STRATEGY 3: Change laws, regulations, and agency practices that have an appreciable but indirect impact on consumer dietary choices so that they make more foods to support nutritionally desirable diets available. Examples are food grading and labeling laws and standards of identity for a number of food products.

ACTION 1: *Improve food labeling and food description, production, and processing regulations to permit consumers to make better informed choices.*

ACTION 2: *Develop and adopt regulations governing food descriptions, grading, and nomenclatural practices.*

ACTION 3: *Improve the nutritional attributes of animal products.*

STRATEGY 4: Enable government feeding facilities to serve as models to private food services and help people meet dietary recommendations.

ACTION 1: *The Office of the Secretary of the U.S. Department of Veterans Affairs should direct its health-care personnel to follow dietary recommendations in all of its food and health care systems.*

ACTION 2: *The surgeons general of the Army, Navy, and Air Force within the Department of Defense (DOD) should develop a plan for implementing dietary recommendations in all aspects of the DOD food and health-care systems.*

ACTION 3: *The DOD's food and beverage services and practices should be revised to conform to dietary recommendations.*

ACTION 4: *Urge the director of the Federal Bureau of Prisons to examine the feasibility of providing diets in line with dietary recommendations, recognizing the complexity of the correctional system and the special role of food in correctional facilities.*

ACTION 5: *The General Services Administration should ensure that food contracts and monitoring systems are made to conform to the principles of dietary recommendations.*

ACTION 6: *Department secretaries should encourage government employees to consume diets that meet dietary recommendations.*

ACTION 7: *The U.S. government personnel ultimately responsible for funding official meal functions should offer meals that are consistent with the principles of dietary recommendations.*

STRATEGY 5: Develop a comprehensive research, monitoring, and evaluation plan to achieve a better understanding of the factors that motivate people to modify their eating habits and to monitor the progress toward implementation of dietary recommendations.

ACTION 1: *The secretaries of USDA and DHHS should mandate increased amounts of intramural research that relate to implementation of dietary recommendations and give high priority to the funding of extramural research in this area.*

ACTION 2: *Improve the National Nutrition Monitoring System and provide it with adequate resources.*

RECOMMENDATIONS TO THE PRIVATE SECTOR

STRATEGY 1: Promote dietary recommendations and motivate consumers to use them in selecting and preparing foods and in developing healthful dietary patterns.

ACTION 1: *Make consumers aware of dietary recommendations and their importance and how available products and services can be used to meet them.*

ACTION 2: *Contribute to efforts to improve the nutrition labeling of food so that it better assists consumers in making informed, nutritionally desirable food choices.*

ACTION 3: *Provide consumers with information at points of purchase so that they may assess quickly some of the nutrition attributes of specific products and brands.*

STRATEGY 2: Continue to increase the availability of a wide variety of appealing foods that help consumers to meet dietary recommendations.

ACTION 1: *Develop more nutritionally desirable products that appeal to consumers.*

ACTION 2: *Contribute to efforts to revise, or develop as appropriate, food-quality criteria (such as standards of identity and grading), pricing structures, and food product descriptors to promote the production of more nutritionally desirable food products.*

ACTION 3: *Engage in practices leading to the greater availability of nutritionally desirable products that will assist consumers in meeting dietary recommendations.*

RECOMMENDATIONS TO HEALTH-CARE PROFESSIONALS

STRATEGY 1: Raise the level of knowledge among all health-care professionals about food and nutrition and the relationships between diet and health.

ACTION 1: *Establish within the faculty of every health-care professional school an identifiable program with overall responsibility for planning and developing a research and education agenda in human nutrition.*

ACTION 2: *Establish a program within the Public Health Service to support the training of faculty in nutrition. The goal should be at least one nutrition faculty member per health-care professional school for each of the licensed graduate programs in the health-care professions.*

ACTION 3: *Materials emphasizing dietary recommendations for students in the health-care professions should be prepared by curriculum committees, authors, publishers, and others with in-*

terests in curriculum development. Such materials should include course syllabi at varying levels of complexity, batteries of examination questions, relevant bibliographic listings, audiovisual teaching instruments, and self-education computer programs.

ACTION 4: *Expand nutrition education of health-care professionals at all levels. Certification and licensing bodies involved in the education of health-care professionals should require a demonstrated knowledge of nutrition.*

STRATEGY 2: Contribute to efforts that will lead to health-promoting dietary changes for health-care professionals, their clients, and the general population.

ACTION 1: *Encourage efforts to implement dietary recommendations in a coordinated manner for maximum effectiveness and to avoid unnecessary duplication.*

ACTION 2: *Encourage all health-care professionals to integrate nutrition information into their multiple counseling, treatment, skills training, and follow-up sessions with individual clients and patients.*

ACTION 3: *Provide leadership, resources, and personnel for the dissemination of sound nutritional advice.*

ACTION 4: *Working as individuals or through professional societies, provide guidance to regulatory and legislative bodies concerned with the establishment of dietary standards and with rules and policies governing the production, harvesting, processing, preservation, distribution, and marketing of food products.*

ACTION 5: *Specialists in human nutrition and food science, working through their professional organizations, should distribute practical information such as menus, recipes, and ideas for health promotion initiatives to private and public providers of meals.*

ACTION 6: *Serve as role models by following dietary recommendations (and practicing other healthy behaviors) as often as possible.*

STRATEGY 3: Intensify research on the relationships between food, nutrition, and health and on the means to use this knowledge to promote the consumption of healthful diets.

ACTION 1: *Encourage sponsors of research to give high priority to research into diet and disease relationships and to developing innovative ways to use that knowledge in educating healthcare professionals and the public about nutrition.*

RECOMMENDATIONS FOR EDUCATION OF THE PUBLIC

STRATEGY 1: Ensure that consistent educational messages about dietary recommendations reach the public.

ACTION 1: *Initiate meetings of leaders and representatives of national groups (e.g., interest groups, professional associations, and Cooperative Extension Service educators) to explore common interests in implementing dietary recommendations and to develop a series of common educational initiatives related to the attainment of that goal.*

ACTION 2: *Review materials on diet and health prepared for the public by various professional groups and organizations to achieve consistency and ensure compatibility with dietary recommendations.*

ACTION 3: *Convene an ad hoc committee composed of authors and publishers of leading nutrition textbooks to develop a series of broad guidelines that publishers could use to provide in their publications consistent and authoritative information on dietary recommendations and their scientific rationale.*

ACTION 4: *Constitute a panel to review and evaluate nutrition education materials made available to schoolteachers from various food industry sources.*

STRATEGY 2: Incorporate principles, concepts, and skills training that support dietary recommendations into all levels of schooling—kindergarten through college.

ACTION 1: *Design a model curriculum for teaching food skills, nutrition, and health from kindergarten through grade 12.*

ACTION 2: *During the development of the curriculum proposed in Action 1, identify teacher-tested lessons—on health, nutrition, and food selection and preparation skills—suitable for use in a variety of classroom settings at different grade levels.*

ACTION 3: *Professional nutrition, health promotion, and education organizations in each state should organize their members (and through their members, local parents) to lobby state legislatures and urge state boards of education to mandate the inclusion of at least one food skills, nutrition, and health course in the requirements for teacher preparation in each state.*

ACTION 4: *Revive, at the level of at least $0.50 per student, the USDA-administered Nutrition Education and Training (NET) Program that stimulated so much activity related to nutrition education in the late 1970s.*

ACTION 5: *Offer a nutrition course or, at a minimum, a life science course with a well-developed nutrition component at institutions of higher learning.*

ACTION 6: *Offer each student in grades 7 through college on a periodic basis (e.g., every 3 years) a computer analysis of his or her diet and a professional evaluation of how the student's food habits conform to dietary recommendations.*

STRATEGY 3: Ensure that children in child-care programs (including out-of-home care programs and family-, group-, or center-based programs) receive nutritious meals served in an environment that takes account of the importance of food in children's physical and emotional well-being.

ACTION 1: *Establish an interdisciplinary task force to oversee food-related matters involving children in child-care programs. This task force would include experts in pediatrics, nutrition, psychology, anthropology, and child development, along with child-care providers and parents.*

ACTION 2: *Public policy committees in nutrition, medical, and other health-related organizations should work to develop and pass legislation to require that foods served to children help them to meet dietary recommendations. The Child and Adult Care Food Program standard of USDA should be used as a quality minimum.*

STRATEGY 4: Enhance consumers' knowledge and the skills they need to meet dietary recommendations through appropriate food selection and preparation.

ACTION 1: *Develop a consumer manual to present strategies that can be used to influence local food providers (and others who play important roles in the food system) to increase the availability of foods that help people meet dietary recommendations.*

ACTION 2: *Prepare an inexpensive, continually updatable foods data bank to inform consumers, food planners, and others about the nutritional content, composition, and production/processing history of the products available to them.*

STRATEGY 5: Establish systems for designing, implementing, and maintaining community-based interventions to improve dietary patterns.

ACTION 1: *Professional organizations concerned with food, nutrition, and health should work to engage community leaders in the development of community-based programs promoting dietary recommendations.*

ACTION 2: *Encourage schools of higher learning in various regions of the country to develop programs for educating and updating individuals in the skills needed to play key roles in community-based nutrition education programs.*

STRATEGY 6: Enlist the mass media to help decrease consumer confusion and increase the knowledge and skills that will motivate and equip consumers to make health-promoting dietary choices.

ACTION 1: *Develop a series of social marketing campaigns to disseminate dietary recommendations.*

ACTION 2: *Appoint a committee of experts in nutrition education, child development, social influence, and media to review past attempts to regulate television food advertising to children.*

ACTION 3: *Appoint a standing committee to coordinate the vast number of media activities necessary to increase consumer knowledge about dietary recommendations and their application and to decrease consumer confusion.*

ACTION 4: *Establish a task force of social scientists to examine the utility of national entertainment television as a community-organizing tool that can be used to enhance efforts of local health agencies in encouraging appropriate dietary changes.*

DIRECTIONS FOR RESEARCH

1. Improve methods to characterize what people actually eat, especially over long periods during which dietary patterns change.
2. Increase understanding of the existing and potential determi-

nants of dietary change and how this knowledge can be used to promote more healthful eating behaviors.

3. Continue research to develop new food products and modify both the production and processing of existing products to help consumers more easily meet dietary recommendations.

4. Review and improve government and private-sector policies that directly and indirectly affect the availability of particular foods and the promotion of healthful dietary patterns.

5. Determine how implementors of dietary recommendations at all levels (e.g., supermarket managers, physicians, and high school health teachers) can more effectively teach the basis of the recommendations and motivate people to follow them.

6. Investigate the costs and benefits of implementing dietary recommendations as proposed by this committee and by others.

Acronyms

AHA	American Heart Association
AOA	Administration on Aging
CDC	Centers for Disease Control
CES	Cooperative Extension Service
DHHS	U.S. Department of Health and Human Services
DOD	Department of Defense
DVA	U.S. Department of Veterans Affairs
EFNEP	Expanded Food and Nutrition Education Program
FDA	Food and Drug Administration
FD&C Act	Food, Drug, and Cosmetic Act
FDPIR	Food Distribution Program on Indian Reservations
FMI	Food Marketing Institute
FNB	Food and Nutrition Board
FNS	Food and Nutrition Service
FSP	Food Stamp Program
FTC	Federal Trade Commission
GAO	U.S. General Accounting Office
GSA	General Services Administration
HNIS	Human Nutrition Information Service
IMPS	Institutional Meat Purchase Specifications
NCEP	National Cholesterol Education Program
NET	Nutrition Education and Training Program
NHANES II	Second National Health and Nutrition Examination Survey, 1976-1980
NHBPEP	National High Blood Pressure Education Program

NHLBI   National Heart, Lung, and Blood Institute
NIH   National Institutes of Health
NRA   National Restaurant Association
PSAs   Public Service Announcements
RDAs   Recommended Dietary Allowances
USDA   U.S. Department of Agriculture
USRDAs   United States Recommended Daily Allowances
WIC   Special Supplemental Food Program for Women, Infants, and Children

Index

industry organizations, 145, 153, 157–
159, 161, 181
milk and milk products, 150–151
prices, 9, 29, 146–147
research, 147, 155, 181, 211–212, 226
travel services, 200
see also Food industry; Food Marketing Institute; Food supply;
Institutional food services; Voluntary organizations and activities
Professional associations, 205
government, relations with, 170,
179–180, 192–193
health care professionals, 97, 109,
123, 179–180, 199–200, 205, 222
industry organizations, 145, 153,
157–159, 161, 181
professional education, 169
promotional campaigns, 12, 148, 149
public information/education, 192–
193, 196, 199–200, 202–203, 205, 225
state-level, 196, 206
see also specific associations
Professional education, 126
food preparation personnel, 14, 123,
125, 132, 159, 161, 162
health care, personnel, 10, 125, 132,
169, 172–174, 175–178, 181, 198,
203, 221–222, 223–224
Nutrition Education and Training
Program, 12, 125, 196–197, 224
nutritionists and dietitians, general,
123, 171–172
teachers, 12, 125, 196, 223–224
Professionals, *see* Nutritionists and
dietitians; Health professionals
Project LEAN, 178, 204
*Promoting Health/Preventing Disease:
Objectives for the Nation*, 19
Protein, 85–86, 101–102, 216
Psychological factors, 5, 23, 28–29, 34
theories, 50–58
see also Attitudes and beliefs;
Preferences; Social influences
Publications, 60, 62, 87, 90, 117, 118–
119, 155, 193, 202
consumer manuals, 97, 200–201, 224
point-of-purchase, 146, 156–157,
159–160, 162, 221
see also Educational materials;
specific published reports
Public education, *see* Elementary and
secondary education

Public Health Service, 10, 176, 221
Public information, 1, 4, 5–6, 8, 11–12,
14–15, 24, 25–26, 42, 90, 144–146,
168, 184–207, 223–225
data banks, 200, 201–202, 225
government role, general, 21, 48–49,
114, 125–126, 219
knowledge *vs* behavior, 14, 16, 22,
40, 47–49, 53–58, 61–62, 190–191
national programs, 29, 113, 178
point-of-purchase, 146, 156–157,
159–160, 162, 201, 203, 221
private sector role, 27, 144–146, 156–
157, 169, 202
professional associations, 192–193,
196, 199–200, 202–203, 205, 225
telephone services, 155, 156, 174, 203
work-site food services, 14, 15, 60,
65, 66–67, 162, 203
see also Advertising; Labeling;
Marketing; Mass media
Public opinion, 6, 168
Public sector, *see* Federal government;
Government role; State goverment
Public service announcements, 26, 205, 206
Public Voice for Food and Health
Policy, 201

Quality control, 135
see also Regulations; Standards
Quantitative guidelines, 20

Recommended Daily Allowances, 191
supplements, 108
Recommended Dietary Allowances, 3,
5– 6, 7, 15, 21, 84–109, 215–217,
220–221, 222
advertising and, 204
information on, general, 11, 197, 200, 201
private sector role, 9, 144–147
research, 16–17
supplements, 216
Regional factors, 158, 225
mass media, 67–68
marketing, 149, 154
professional education, 203
Regulations, 1, 7, 13, 27, 127–130, 200, 219
advertising, 188–190, 204, 225
Agriculture Department, 93, 121–
123, 128, 130, 186, 190, 219
childhood nutrition, 12, 188
federal, general, 93, 121–124, 128–
130, 133–134, 185–186, 218–219; *see*

F

REC'

REC'D JI